Conducting Psychiatric Consultations

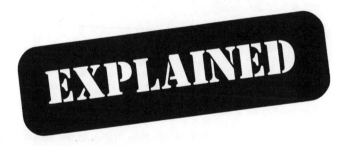

EXPLAINED

David J. Robinson, M.D., F.R.C.P.C.
Diplomate of the American Board of Psychiatry & Neurology

Rapid Psychler Press

Suite 374
3560 Pine Grove Ave.
Port Huron, Michigan
USA 48060

Suite 203
1673 Richmond St.
London, Ontario
Canada N6G 2N3

Toll-Free Phone 888-PSY-CHLE (888-779-2453)
Toll-Free Fax   888-PSY-CHLR (888-779-2457)
Outside the U.S. & Canada — Fax 519-675-0610
website www.psychler.com
email   rapid@psychler.com

ISBN 1-894328-22-1
Printed in the United States of America
© 2000, Rapid Psychler Press
First Edition, First Printing

Dedication

This book is dedicated to my friend (and keen-eyed proof reader)

Tom Norry, B.Sc.N.

Acknowledgments

I am indebted to the following individuals for their unfailing support in assisting me with this text.

- **Brian & Fanny Chapman**
- **Monty & Lil Robinson**
- **Lisa & Cathy Burgard**
- **Nicole & Mark Kennedy**
- **Dr. Donna Robinson & Dr. Robert Bauer**
- **Dean Avola**
- **Brad Groshok**

I would also like to thank the following people for their helpful reviews of this manuscript.

- **Paul I. Steinberg, M.D.**
- **Tom Norry, B.Sc.N.**
- **Philip Jones, M.D.**
- **Thomas Gantert, B.Sc.N.**
- **Lisa & Cathy Burgard**
- **Dr. Sandra Northcott**
- **Dr. Lisa Bogue**
- **Dr. Michelle Kelly**

Rapid Psychler Press

produces books and presentation media that are:
• comprehensively researched
• well organized
• formatted for ease of use
• reasonably priced
• clinically oriented, and
• include humor that enhances education, and that neither demeans patients nor the efforts of those who treat them

Table of Contents

Publication Notes

Terminology
Throughout this book, the term "patient" refers to people who are suffering and seek help. The term further describes those who bear pain without complaint or anger. The terms "consumer" or "consumer-survivor" reflect an unfortunate trend that is pejorative towards mental health care, labeling it as if it were a trade or business instead of a profession. These terms are also ambiguous, as it is not clear what is being "consumed" or "survived."

Graphics
All of the illustrations in this book are original works of art commissioned by Rapid Psychler Press and are a signature feature of our publications. Rapid Psychler Press makes available an entire library of color illustrations (including those from this book) as 35mm slides and overhead transparencies. These images are available for viewing and can be purchased from our website — **www.psychler.com**

These images from our color library may be used for presentations. We request that you respect our copyright and do not reproduce these images in any form for any purpose at any time.

Bolded Terms
Throughout this book, various terms appear in bolded text which allows for ease of identification. Many of these terms are defined in this text. Some, however, are only mentioned because a detailed description is beyond the scope of this book. Fuller explanations of all of the bolded terms can be found in standard reference texts.

1/ Introduction to C-L Psychiatry

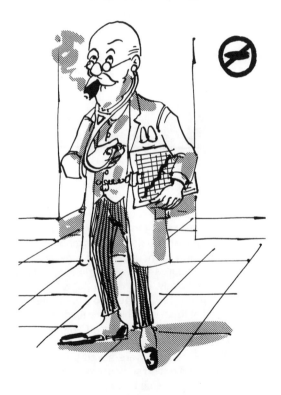

What is Consultation-Liaison Psychiatry?

Consultation-Liaison (C-L) refers to the branch or subspecialty of psychiatry that focuses on the interface between psychological (mental) and somatic (medical) illnesses.

The main function of C-L psychiatry is to provide clinical services that link mental health professionals to those in other medical specialties (as illustrated below), on both an inpatient and outpatient basis. C-L psychiatry also has education and research components.

C-L psychiatry can be conceptualized as bridging the gap between illnesses which are entirely physical in nature and those considered to have entirely psychological causes.

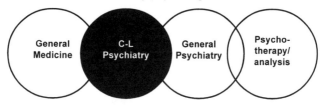

Depending on the availability of clinical resources, some hospitals have psychiatrists who further specialize and offer their services exclusively to areas where the psychosocial aspects of illness are particularly pronounced. The most common services requiring this degree of psychiatric involvement are: Transplantation, Cardiology, Gastroenterology, Oncology, and HIV Clinics. Thompson (1993) contacted 210 psychiatrists selected by him. Half of them were prominent educators and/ or clinicians who did not primarily practice C-L psychiatry, and the other half were from the **Academy of Psychosomatic Medicine (APM)**. Recipients were asked to define the role, patient population, and expertise possessed by C-L psychiatrists. Their consensus was as follows:

Introduction to C-L Psychiatry

C-L psychiatrists evaluate and treat inpatients and outpatients with significant medical and surgical illness who are also experiencing significant psychiatric symptoms. These patients' symptoms may be due to their medical-surgical conditions, medical-surgical medications, and other treatments (and may be worsened by these factors), and their psychiatric symptoms may be interfering with optimal medical management.

Who Practices C-L Psychiatry?

Noyes (1992) reported on the APM survey of the 6000 members of the **American Psychiatric Association (APA)** who indicated an interest in C-L psychiatry. It was estimated that about 7.5% of psychiatrists spent at least one-quarter of their time engaged in C-L work, and nearly 3.2% spent at least half their time doing so. The majority of psychiatrists conducted less than 150 inpatient consults per year, though some were referred up to 600. About 10.5% of the APA membership had some affiliation with a C-L service (i.e. are involved in conducting consults, educational activities or research).

C-L is the Complete Subspecialty

Psychiatry is a diverse field. Psychiatrists are often unfortunately polarized into being either principally psychopharmacologists (biologically oriented) or psychotherapists (dynamically oriented). Both sides have their strengths and weaknesses, proponents and opponents. There are subspecialties within psychiatry that further define the range of patients that some psychiatrists treat. Though all psychiatrists complete medical school, the knowledge they acquired often plays a minimal role in their day-to-day work. C-L is the subspecialty that ties together all the "factions" of psychiatry, as well as keeping its practitioners in touch with medical and surgical practices. C-L psychiatrists require at least a working knowledge of the following areas:

9

- Psychotherapy
- Forensics
- Addictions
- Neuropsychiatry

- Psychopharmacology
- Geriatric & Adolescent Psychiatry
- Emergency Psychiatry
- Crisis Intervention

In this way, C-L psychiatry is the complete subspecialty. The diagnostic diversity is at least as varied as that encountered on general psychiatry units, with additional skills being required to adapt management plans to patients' physical illnesses.

Since the majority of psychiatrists engaged in C-L work do not make this their only avenue of practice, they have the opportunity to enhance their skills in other areas. It is not unusual to have researchers, psychoanalysts or even administrative psychiatrists involved in C-L activities for a portion of their practice.

Langlsey (1988) conducted a survey among psychiatric practitioners and educators regarding their opinions on what skills and knowledge define a specialist in psychiatry. Forty-eight items regarding skills and fifty-one items regarding knowledge were ranked. Those particularly relevant to C-L psychiatry with an agreement of at least 90% are listed below with their rank:

Rank	Skill
1	• Conduct a comprehensive diagnostic interview
10	• Maintain records including history, mental status exam, physical examination, diagnostic tests, and progress notes
11	• Conduct crisis intervention
12	• Use appropriate laboratory tests, psychological testing, and other diagnostic procedures
14	• Conduct a comprehensive assessment and develop a management plan for physically or psycho-somatically ill patients

15   • Conduct brief psychotherapy
16   • Develop liaison relationships with other professionals

Rank   Knowledge
2   • Differentiate between physical and psychiatric disorders
5   • Evaluation and management of psychiatric emergencies
11   • Psychiatrically relevant aspects of neurology
12   • Psychological aspects of stress, coping, loss, bereavement, etc.
13   • Syndromes of importance in C-L psychiatry
14   • Indications/contraindications for various forms of psychotherapy

C-L work requires the greatest breadth of skill and knowledge of all the areas in psychiatry. As an example, consider the range of abilities required to manage the following case:

A sixty-seven year old male with a history of bipolar mood disorder is admitted after a lithium overdose. Because of his high serum lithium level, he is too obtunded to consent to dialysis, which is deemed necessary by the medical consultant. Substitute consent is obtained for this procedure. After recovering from the overdose, he goes into alcohol withdrawal delirium two days later and attempts to leave hospital.

After crisis intervention takes place to prevent him from leaving, his status is changed to that of an involuntary patient (due to safety concerns and so he can receive further treatment). He receives medication to treat his withdrawal. Once he recovers from the withdrawal delirium, he requests psychotherapy to help him deal with his "anniversary reaction" to his wife's death.

Abilities & Skills of a C-L Psychiatrist

• Has an expert knowledge of psychiatric disorders, a working knowledge of medical (physical) disorders, and the ability to understand the relationship between the two (**biopsychosocial** orientation)

• Able to use varied treatment modalities for medically ill patients (especially in psychopharmacology); provision of short-term psychotherapy is an important aspect of care that was not initially emphasized in early concepts of C-L service

• Capable of communicating with physicians, housestaff, nurses, and patients in a non-psychiatric environment

• Able to discern and accommodate the idiosyncrasies of consultees and specialized units; observant of both the needs of the consultee and the patient; able to respond to all parties in a beneficial manner

• Able to gather clinical data from several sources into a coherent summary (formulation) using a biopsychosocial approach to develop and implement a management plan

• Able to rapidly obtain and assimilate information, form hypotheses, and make effective interventions; these skills may differ from those required in other areas of psychiatry

• Able to elicit pathological findings/ diagnostic criteria in interviews and **mental status examinations (MSE)**

• Cognizant of the legal and ethical principles involved in patients' medical care (e.g. competence to consent to treatment, confidentiality, sharing of records, etc.)

• Able to interpret basic hematologic, biochemical, and

neuroimaging results, and be knowledgeable in directing further testing (for both medical and psychological aspects)

• Being an interested teacher who is capable of passing along useful information to referring sources as well as teaching nurses, students, psychologists, social workers, etc., and leading a multidisciplinary team

Qualities of a C-L Psychiatrist

• Able to wait for others to recognize problems that were potentially obvious at an earlier point (and then await the consult request)

• Able to tolerate abuse and rejection from patients who are not cooperative or haven't been informed of consults

• Able to admit he or she doesn't know what is wrong and/ or has little (or nothing) to offer

• Able to tolerate not getting paid for some clinical work

• Avoid pretending to be able to magically treat the patient

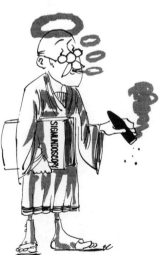

• Constantly monitors management steps and changes approaches quickly when they are not successful

• Able to tolerate criticisms of the specialty (valid or not)

• Able to tolerate disruptions and keep a flexible schedule

Consultation Psychiatry

Although the term **C-L** is usually globally applied to the activities described above, **consultation** and **liaison** in practice encompass separate functions.

Consultation refers to the provision of clinical services for a patient at the request of the primary (non-psychiatric) physician. The consultation involves an interview, followed by the development and implementation of a treatment plan. The aim of the consultation is to answer the clinical question(s) posed by the referring physician, and to assist in the management of this central problem and related issues. The consultation model requires the consultee to initiate the process. Requests are made once problems have developed and have been recognized. In this way, the consultations focus on **secondary prevention** (limiting the development of symptoms after they have developed) and **tertiary prevention** (rehabilitating patients to prevent the recurrence of symptoms). There is no structured teaching of psychiatric principles, though clinical points germane to the particular case may be emphasized. Consultation services meet the basic clinical needs of referring sources.

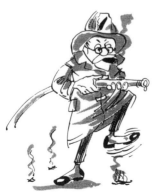

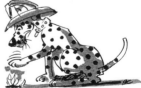

A frequent comparison of the consultation model is that of "putting out fires."

Liaison Psychiatry

Liaison (a French term meaning "to bind") was first used by Billings in 1939, and refers to activities that promote an awareness of psychiatric and psychosocial issues in patients' care. These educational contacts can be either formal (e.g. structured teaching rounds) or informal, and are carried out to:

• Increase the attention paid to the psychosocial aspects of a patient's care and to practice **primary prevention** strategies (preventing the development of psychological symptoms)
• Educate medical/surgical colleagues about the psychological effects of being ill, and how this affects recovery
• Impart basic psychosocial knowledge and help foster the ability of other physicians in detection and triage techniques
• Provide continuing education for non-psychiatrists, and to promote structural changes in medical/surgical settings

Liaison psychiatrists do not wait for formal consults to be requested — they involve themselves in the care of patients on a particular service where significant psychiatric issues are identified. Formal teaching is provided in areas relevant to patients' needs. Education of patients and families regarding psychosocial issues is another commonly requested liaison activity.

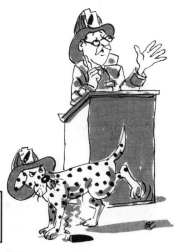

A frequent comparison of the liaison model is that of lecturing on fire safety.

Despite the gains that can be made in both patient care and educating physicians, liaison activities have generally been declining since the 1980's, mainly due to funding difficulties. Rosenbaum & McCarty (1994) explained the fate of liaison psychiatry in terms of the milieu on medical/ surgical wards. In these areas, physicians face the following challenges:

• Acquiring and mastering the skills in their own disciplines
• Looking after seriously ill patients
• Providing care primarily to reduce symptoms
• Facilitating discharge from the hospital in a timely manner

Medical and surgical residents are just as humane as psychiatric residents, however, given the highly demanding circumstances of their training, it may be adaptive to suppress humanistic interests (at particular times). Though few hospital psychiatry departments offer liaison services, consultation activities can still provide a comprehensive range of services.

References

D.G. Langsley & J. Yager
The Definition of a Psychiatrist: Eight Years Later
American Journal of Psychiatry 145: p. 469 — 475, 1988

R. Noyes Jr., T. Wise & J. Hayes
Consultation-Liaison Psychiatrists: How Many Are There and How Are They Funded?
Psychosomatics 33(2): p. 123 — 127, 1992

M. Rosenbaum & T. McCarty
The Relationship of Psychosomatic Medicine to Consultation-Liaison Psychiatry
Psychosomatics 35(6): p. 569 — 573, 1994

T.L. Thompson II
Should We Shift the Name for "Consultation-Liaison" to "Medical-Surgical" Psychiatry, "Psychiatry in Medicine and Surgery," or Some Other Term?
Psychosomatics 34(3): p. 259 — 264, 1993

2/ Conducting the Consultation

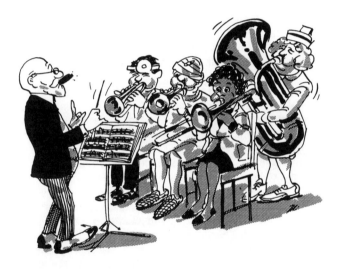

The next three chapters provide an overview on performing a psychiatric consultation which involves the following steps:

- **Receiving the Referral**
- **Preparing for the Consult**
- **Interviewing the Patient**
- **Writing the Consultation Report** (Ch. 3)
- **Implementing the Treatment Plan** (Ch. 4)

Consultation requests are initiated by phone, letter or personal contact. Keeping a central registry of medical and demographic information is frequently done and helpful for a variety of clinical, administrative and research purposes.

It is a common occurrence for other services to ask for an informal consultation (often called a "curbside"). This may be appropriate between consultants or in a non-teaching center, but has significant disadvantages for students and residents. The experience of performing a complete consult is lost, as is the opportunity of offering more to the patient than simply answering a clinical question or two. Each supervisor will have his or her own policy and rationale, but in general it is not good clinical practice to reduce a consultation to a single clinical point without the benefit of more information or interviewing the patient. For example, you are asked, "Which antipsychotic has strong sedative properties? This can become a medicolegal issue if you unwittingly suggest chlorpromazine for a patient who has a pre-existing seizure disorder that you weren't told about at the time.

Receiving the Referral

Many centers have preprinted forms for recording both consult requests and the actual consultations. If some demographic information isn't provided initially, it can be added after the consult has been completed. Having as much data as possible beforehand increases the effectiveness of your preparation and interview.

The following mnemonic summarizes the essential information to record when a consult is requested:

"I'M SURE"

Identifying factors (name, age, gender, marital status, race, religion, occupation, etc.)

Medical problem(s)

Source of referral (referring physician and service)

Urgency (routine, urgent, emergency)

Reason for referral

Expectations of the consultee

The **identifying factors**, as in any medical document, help develop a picture of the patient. Each factor has its own clinical implications and helps tailor your preparation for the consult. These factors also have the practical advantage of helping you to recognize the patient on a busy medical or surgical ward. You may well pass the person in the hallway or need to identify him or her in a room of several people.

An awareness of the patient's **medical problem** is valuable to have before the consult. This helps keep your general medical knowledge current. Also, discussing the medical situation is a good way of initiating a consult interview.

Knowing the **source** of the referral also helps with particular aspects of the consult. Different services and referring physicians have expectations and idiosyncrasies that, once understood, make the process easier and more effective. Aspects such as the protocol for having investigations and treatment suggestions approved, or the degree of detail expected, vary considerably between referring sources.

It is crucial to clarify the **urgency** of the consult. Most C-L services have a time frame for inpatient and outpatient assessments (e.g. twenty-four hours, and three days respectively). It is good practice to inform the consultee approximately when to expect your visit. Urgent consults often need to be seen the morning or afternoon in which they are requested. Emergencies are usually relayed from consultant to consultant. For such occasions, it is helpful to have the following available:

> • A crisis team with physical and chemical restraints
> • A knowledge of the laws in your area regarding involuntary committal, rights advice, and medicolegal forms
> • Phone numbers for the police and hospital security
> • Familiarity with non-violent crisis intervention

In general, all consults should be seen as soon as possible. The referring source has come to a point where your expertise and input are necessary. Prompt attention will be appreciated and reciprocated when you request consults. Simply performing the consult can be of benefit to the patient and referring team. For example:

> • Conducting the consult tells the patient that his or her problems have been heard and acted upon; many medical and surgical units are so busy that they do not have the time to explore psychosocial problems
> • Your investigations may reveal added biological precipitants or perpetuating factors

• In appropriate cases, transfer to the psychiatry unit puts the patient in a more suitable milieu and frees up a bed (for which you should expect enduring gratitude)

Some unpleasant events can occur if the consult is delayed:

• The patient may be discharged or may die
• The physician may change his or her mind
• The patient may decline the consult
• The clinical condition can worsen

The crux of the consult is of course the **reason for referral**. This becomes "the question" that has to be answered at the end of the assessment. Page twenty-four lists the most common reasons for which psychiatric consults are requested.

What If No Reason For Referral Is Given?
Despite the integral role the consult question plays, it is surprising how often it is omitted from the request. This is perhaps the reason why "consults" are sometimes sarcastically referred to as "insults." The consultee has obviously come to a point where he or she requests help for a patient's psychiatric problem, but may have trouble expressing a clear reason for the referral.

Some psychiatrists refuse to see consults until all of the preliminary information is provided. This approach may be gratifying for the egos of such individuals, and may have merit in that these clinicians are somewhat more fully informed before seeing the patient. However, this approach fails to consider that a vague or absent "reason" often indicates that a greater degree of assistance is needed, and that the psychiatric problem may be of a more serious nature (Golinger, 1985). Additionally, it can force the consultee into putting "something" down on the request to impel such consultants to see the patient. Even with straightforward cases, the reason listed on the consult form may not ultimately be the area of greatest importance. This has been aptly described by Schiff & Pilot (1959) who stated that psychiatric consultations. . . *stem from the referring physician's concerns, of which the most cogent are frequently not stated.* Lipowski (1967) added that. . . *the request may bear little relevance to the real nature of the problem, and that the more diffuse and unclear the message, the more likely the consultee is in need of assistance.*

Some primary physicians will refer patients because they are not well acquainted with psychiatric problems. In other situations, it may be that serious psychiatric illnesses engender confusion and anxiety among referring physicians. The tolerance for disturbing or disruptive behaviors may be fairly low on medical/surgical units, especially with problems such as:

- Noncompliance with medications or procedures
- Wandering, agitated or highly vocal patients
- Suicidal thoughts or gestures
- Expression of strong affect

Some physicians grudgingly make referrals (and some make none at all) because to them it is an admission of not being "omniscient and omnipotent." Furthermore, it can be demoralizing to insist that referring physicians append consult requests before patients will be seen (perhaps to the point where no request is made). In spite of the ultimate quality of your assessment, these preliminary matters can have an overriding effect on the whole consult (even an excellent consult may not restore rapport with an irritated referring physician).

Psychiatrists are among the physicians least likely to make consult requests, and may well perform less of a work-up for referrals than other services. For example, a referral to a cardiologist for an "abnormal heart rhythm" will often suffice. Having to further specify the type of arrhythmia and provide a preliminary interpretation of an EKG is beyond the expectations of a psychiatric service. It is beneficial to bear this in mind for the referrals you receive. Consult requests sent to psychiatrists are in general at least as well documented as referrals between other specialties, and may contain more information.

Keep in mind that a vaguely worded reason for referral may well mean the presence of a serious psychiatric illness, and that even a clearly stated one may not be accurate. It is more the responsibility of C-L psychiatry to effectively manage patients than it is to educate our colleagues, especially on how to make "proper" referrals. A number of authors have investigated the resistance to requesting consultations shown by non-psychiatric physicians. While the comparative ranking of different reasons varies between reports, the factors described were relatively similar:

Patient-Related
• Patient's reaction is expectable based on his or her illness
• Relationship with the patient may be harmed by the referral
• Don't wish to deal with the issues brought about by the consult
• Poor past experience with a psychiatrist
• Don't want to "lose" patient to another physician

Psychiatrist-Related
• Don't have faith in psychiatry
• Don't believe a psychiatrist will help this particular problem
• primary physician should be able to handle the problem
• Poor access to a psychiatrist
• Cost of consult is too high — a social worker or psychologist can perform the same service for less
• Wish to avoid having potential deficits in management highlighted
• Don't want to have deficits in knowledge made obvious
• Psychiatrists infrequently keep physicians informed about patients' progress

Common Consultation Requests

Consults are most commonly requested for the following reasons:

Affect or Mood Changes

• Depression, anxiety, hostility, irritability, euphoria, etc.

Behavioral Problems

• Agitation or impulsivity; aggression towards self or others
• Demanding to leave the unit; refusing treatment
• Crisis intervention (non-violent); chemical or physical restraint

Capacity Determinations and Forensic Issues

• Capacity consent to treatment (informed consent)
• Ability to manage finances or make a Will (**testamentary capacity**)
• Involuntary hospitalization
• Ethical issues

Coping With Medical Illness

• Difficulty accepting diagnosis and/or treatment
• Psychological Factors Affecting Medical Conditions (**PFAMC**)
• Issues regarding terminal illness (e.g. pain, bereavement, dying, etc.)
• Maladaptive reaction to illness (e.g. excessive denial, counterphobic attitude, acute stress disorder, posttraumatic stress disorder)
• Difficulty interacting with staff members

Diagnostic Evaluation

- Veracity of complaints (e.g. investigate the possibility of factitious disorder, malingering or a somatoform disorder)
- Diagnostic evaluation of psychological complaints

Factors Related to Personal or Psychiatric History

- Sexual abuse; child abuse; elder abuse
- Personality disorders
- Substance use disorder
- Monitoring patients with pre-existing psychiatric disorders even if there are no acute issues (i.e. increasing consultees' comfort level)

Mental Status Changes

- Delirium, dementia, psychosis, etc.

Treatment

- Psychotherapy, pharmacology or other (e.g. ECT)
- Transfer of care to an inpatient unit or outpatient program (e.g. resuscitated and detoxified after an overdose)

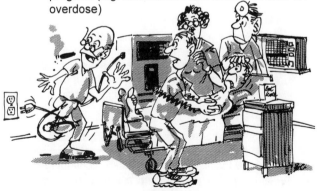

Along with the reason for the referral, the consultee often specifies **expectations** for the consult. Some centers include this as an additional check-box on consult forms. This is usually one of the following three possibilities:

❐ Please see and advise
❐ Please see and transfer care
❐ Please see and follow

The first option most commonly occurs in the following situations:

• Starting, stopping or switching medications
• Diagnostic clarification (including an opinion on whether or not a psychiatric illness is present)
• The patient is due to be discharged
• To arrange outpatient follow-up

The second option is usually requested in the following circumstances:

• Patients who are "medically cleared" but have persisting psychiatric illnesses or ongoing suicidal ideation
• A locked unit or constant observation is needed for reasons of elopement or suicidal/homicidal ideation
• Patients whose psychiatric illness poses more of a treatment concern than does the medical condition, and who can be managed medically if the referring source continues to follow the patient on the psychiatry unit

The most common arrangement involves a consult with follow-up visits provided for the duration of the admission. Even in cases where this isn't explicitly stated, continuing contact is appreciated and is good medical practice. The vast majority of studies reporting the benefits and positive impact of psychiatric consultations are based on assessments accompanied by ongoing visits. The usefulness of one-time only consultations is less clear, and intuitively this would seem to make a smaller impact because less time and effort has been devoted to determining the problem and helping the patient. Continuing to provide follow-up care has several advantages:

- Additional history can be obtained from the patient
- Assessing the day-to-day developments (e.g. **Mini-Mental State Exam (MMSE)** scores in a delirious patient)
- Refining your diagnostic impression
- Monitoring the effectiveness of your treatment suggestions and being able to adjust them as the need arises
- Providing other consultation services beyond the one(s) requested (e.g. assessing financial competence)
- Advising on the need or suitability of psychiatric care after discharge

Medical and surgical units are busy places. Rounds may be held early enough in the day that some patients are still asleep. Teaching seminars, procedures, new admissions, documentation, reading up on current cases, and exam preparation all take time away from direct patient contact. Being in hospital becomes even more discouraging when people miss their doctors during rounds and wait for hours to get the chance to have their questions answered.

Psychiatric consultation staff often have the advantage of being able to spend longer periods of time with patients at flexible intervals. By seeing patients regularly, and at times other than morning or afternoon team rounds, you have the opportunity to become important figures in patients' treatment.

In using a "holistic" biopsychosocial approach, C-L service providers may well be the first or only ones to ask about certain aspects of patients' lives. All illnesses make an impact on patients' ability to function in social and occupational roles, which are areas our colleagues do not always have time to explore. We are also the most appropriate ones to assess the effectiveness of our treatment suggestions. For example, psychiatric C-L staff would be aware that antidepressants often treat the symptoms of depression in a predictable sequence and can document changes in mood, cognitive, and vegetative signs instead of globally stating that someone "looks less depressed today."

Preparing for the Consult

Depending on factors such as level of training, supervisor's preferences, idiosyncrasies of the referring source, nature of the consult, and knowledge of the medical problem, some preparation may be required before interviewing the patient. This process can be seen as an interaction between four entities:

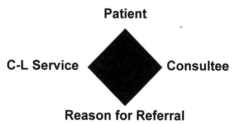

Patient

C-L Service   **Consultee**

Reason for Referral

Each of these four factors contributes to the success of individual referrals and the ongoing usefulness of a C-L Service. If there isn't an understanding of, and balance between these factors, the consultation process can become unsatisfactory in any number of ways. For example:

1. The C-L resident makes an accurate diagnosis and initiates an effective treatment plan, but waited two days to see the patient when an urgent request was made.

2. The referring source neglects to authorize a suggested medication because a case report warns of the possibility of a (rare) complication. While the patient is willing to try the drug, the referring physician does not wish to take even a calculated risk.

3. In order to appease the C-L supervisor and the referring physician, a resident stays late to see a new referral. While the interview is complete, the resident is curt with the patient and takes shortcuts in writing the consult report (due to the late hour).

C-L Service expectations can and should be outlined at the beginning of a rotation. Experience with referring sources and dealing with a variety of problems provides the expertise for these aspects of the consult. Patient factors are always individual and can only be elucidated at the time of the consult.

C-L Service Parameters

• Does the supervisor want to review all consults before they are seen? Only after they are seen? On a case-by-case basis?
• How quickly should consults be seen?
• How soon is the supervisor available to review new consults?
• Are there some treatments that can be started without direct supervision based on the residents' expertise?
• What is expected in terms of documentation? (e.g. are notes to be written or dictated, length of notes)

Consultee Parameters

- Can orders be written directly, or do they need to be co-signed by the C-L supervisor and/or physician?
- Is there an expectation for references (articles) to be provided with consults? (if so, how often and how many?)
- How likely is the consultee to implement suggestions? Does this vary for recommendations made for investigations, medications or psychotherapy?
- How much documentation does the referring source expect?
- How interested is the consultee in learning about psychiatry? How much of an explanation for recommendations is required or desired?

Reason for Referral

- If another avenue becomes important to pursue, does the consultee have to give prior approval? (e.g. an initial request asks for sedation for a behaviorally disturbed patient, but the need arises to assess the person's capacity to consent to medical treatment)
- Should consultees who habitually provide scant documentation or unclear reasons for consultation be targeted for discussions to remedy this?

Patient Parameters

- Was the patient informed of the consult?
- Did the patient request the consult? To what extent does the patient desire the consult?
- Has the person seen a psychiatrist or other mental health professional before?
- Can the patient currently participate in an interview?

Touching base with a supervisor prior to the interview can be of practical assistance. The following examples illustrate how experience can help fine tune a consult.

- "Dr. Flannelette always gives blanket approval to our suggestions."
- "Our inpatient ward is full at the moment, so don't make any commitments about a transfer to Dr. Turf."
- "Dr. Crunch makes referrals at the last moment."
- "Speak to Dr. Nightingale's nurse before doing anything."

Chart Review

The following areas are of special significance in consultation psychiatry and need to be reviewed before seeing the patient.

Hospitalization Particulars
- Length of hospital stay prior to the consult request?
- How did the patient come to medical attention?

Medical/ Surgical History
- Type, course, and severity of the illness
- Treatments currently being used and their efficacy
- Plans for future investigations and treatment
- What has the patient been told about his or her condition and prognosis?

History of the Reasons for the Consultation
- Precipitating and perpetuating factors
- Exacerbations and remissions of behavioral problems
- Possible association of changes in mental status with procedures, interventions, medications, etc.
- Was anything brought in by visitors? (e.g. ethanol, pills from home, food, etc.)

Medication Review
> • Psychiatric complications of non-psychiatric medications (e.g. steroids, antihypertensives)
> • Pre-existing conditions made worse, or new medical problems caused by psychiatric medications

Laboratory Investigation Review
> • Has appropriate testing been carried out, and have the results been reported?
> • Have levels been drawn for applicable medications?
> • Is there an association between biochemical or hematologic abnormalities and altered mental status?

Review of Information
> • Check the emergency record and all multidisciplinary notes to obtain or corroborate information
> • peruse old charts for relevant history

Other Preparation

There are two other aspects that need to be attended to for the consult to occur smoothly and in a time-efficient manner.

Contact the Ward

With the increased emphasis on shortening the length of hospitalization, inpatient stays can involve one procedure after another. Calling ahead to ask about the patient's whereabouts and scheduling a time for the interview can save you a trip.

If the patient is off the floor, ask if a test is being done. This can help you gauge a time to return to the ward. Consults can also be performed in waiting areas (if suitable).

Patients may not speak English fluently. Interpreters can be arranged which is preferable to using family members for this role.

Brush up on the Medical/ Surgical Problem
The patient's illness will have a large bearing on the consult. Your understanding of this illness is paramount to understanding the person and the difficulties he or she is experiencing.

Part of the subspecialty of C-L psychiatry involves knowing which illnesses and medications can precipitate or perpetuate changes in mental status. This requires a working knowledge (and frequent review) of physical medicine. This basis can also be helpful in the "detective work" of the consult. For example, in knowing that intravenous benzodiazepines are given for some procedures, you can make sense of an episode of disinhibited behavior.

One of the best ways of initiating a consult interview is to ask about the patient's illness, treatment, etc. Speaking knowledgeably about this establishes you as an expert and builds a common ground for you to then branch out into a more detailed psychiatric inquiry. Approaches to initiating the consult are provided later in this chapter.

Interviewing the Patient

Usually the most common obstacle in conducting consults is that the patient hasn't been informed of your visit. Mental illness still carries a stigma in society, which unfortunately continues to extend to the hospital staff as well as the lay public.

This lack of notifying patients occurs so frequently that it has been the subject of a paper by Bagheri (1981). This study found that 68% of patients were not told that a psychiatric referral had been made. There was no correlation found between the rank or specialty of the referring physician and the likelihood of informing the patient.

The patient's medical/ psychiatric problem seemed to have a

bearing on the process of notification. Patients with personality or adjustment disorders were more likely to be told than those with psychotic disorders or organic brain syndromes.

Next, the authors asked referring physicians why they hadn't informed patients, and in a separate questionnaire, why they thought their colleagues might not do so. The results are as follows:

Reasons why referring physicians didn't inform patients (ranked from the most to the least common):

- Didn't think of it
- Too busy
- Thought the patient wouldn't understand
- Thought someone else had done it
- Feared the patient might be offended

Reasons why physicians thought others making psychiatric referrals don't inform patients (from most to least common):

- Patients would be insulted and become upset
- The consult might be refused by the patient
- It might damage rapport with referring physician
- The physician was too busy

Referring physicians may choose not to inform patients about consults as a means of coping with their own ambivalence about the referral, or psychiatry in general. Another major factor is the fear of offending patients to the point of damaging rapport.

A study by Steinberg (1980) investigated the veracity of physicians' fears in not making referrals. Fifty patients, who had not originally been referred, had their charts reviewed regarding the suitability for a consultation. On this basis a consult was recommended, and agreed to, in twenty-nine cases. Of these, twenty-one were very receptive to the referral and five were deemed neutral. Wise (1985) found over 80% of patients accepted consults favorably. Despite physicians' reluctance, the great majority of patients view the intervention as positive.

It remains important to realize that a spectrum of attitudes towards psychiatry exists among our colleagues. Whether they are rationalizing their own reasons for not informing patients (e.g. too busy, someone else did it), or projecting their concerns onto patients (e.g. ruining rapport), it is a cogent point to keep in mind that many, if not the majority, of potential referrals aren't made.

Approaches to Initiating the Consult

It is helpful to personally contact the referring source prior to the consult for the following reasons:

> • To obtain information not provided with the request
> • To clarify/ verify expectations
> • To get a last-minute update on the patient's condition

As outlined, you will be speaking to patients who, in the majority of cases, don't know about the consult. You can use the pre-consult contact (meeting or phone call) with the referring source as an opportunity to ask if notification was given, and whether the physician will introduce you to the patient. This is ideal because it introduces the patient to a team/ multidisciplinary approach to treatment. The introduction can benefit, rather than harm, the relationship between the patient and the referring physician. Reluctant consultees can be told about the benefits of a personal introduction. These are that:

- It indicates a mutual awareness that there is an emotional or psychiatric problem
- It demonstrates a willingness on the physician's part to arrange for the expertise needed to help
- It relieves primary physicians of having to deal with certain aspects of patients' care, and allows them to focus on their areas of expertise by identifying someone who will deal with these issues
- The clear majority of patients are receptive to psychiatric consultations

Some C-L psychiatrists expect that patients haven't been told about the referral and just see patients directly. Some will ask if an introduction can be made, but not insist on this. Others will not start the interview until the consultee accompanies them to see the patient. Again, while there is merit to each approach, it is important to keep in mind that referring physicians have reasons for not informing patients about visits from psychiatrists, and this too must be considered, and respected, in the overall consultation process. Ideally, an introduction to patients is made by the referring physician:

> **Physician:** "Mr. XYY, we've spoken previously about your aggressive demeanor on this unit. I've asked one of my colleagues to speak with you to help out with this problem. This is Dr. Eager, he is a resident from the Department of Psychiatry."
> **Dr. Eager:** "Good morning, Mr. XYY. Are you feeling up to speaking with me right now?"
> **Mr. XYY:** "Absolutely, Dr. Eager."
> **Physician:** "Very well. I'll leave you to talk."

More frequently, however, the C-L psychiatrist must independently inform patients that a consult has been requested. This creates two difficulties, first introducing the idea of the consult, and second that it is to occur at that moment.

In most cases, medical and surgical wards have rooms for one, two or four patients (called private, semi-private and quad/ward rooms, respectively). While patients generally are receptive to psychiatric consults, they are often less keen about their roommates knowing that one has been arranged.

Here are some suggestions for approaching this problem.

> • Have someone (usually the patient's nurse) take him or her to a private interview room
> • Introduce yourself as part of the medical or surgical team and ask if the patient would be agreeable to speaking in private where you can then give a fuller explanation
> • Speak in a hushed manner to preclude others from listening to your introduction
> • Ask the others in the room to step out for your interview (if this is reasonable and practical)
> • Introduce yourself as a psychiatric consultant and offer to conduct the interview elsewhere or at another time (which at least preserves confidentiality)

Outline of the C-L Interview

The C-L interview has some unique qualities that sets it apart from a general psychiatric interview.

For many patients, this is their first contact with a psychiatrist, or likely, any mental health professional. They usually have not been informed of your visit, may not agree with it, or see the rationale for why it was requested.

Patients won't know what is expected of them. They may only know about psychiatrists from their friends or the media. Jokes about mental illnesses are common, with references pervading many conversations. For example:

- "You've been acting kind of psychotic lately."
- "My supervisor has really lost his mind this time."
- "The voice in my head tells me to take a vacation."

While the patient's friends and family may, in the past, have been teasing about his or her need to see a psychiatrist, finally meeting one is still another matter.

In contrast to some other types of psychiatric interviews, the C-L interview is usually quite active and engaging. An explanation detailing your position in the hospital and interest/ expertise in psychiatry is frequently appropriate and helpful. A large number of people can be involved in a patient's care on medical/surgical units. A detailed introduction is welcome, as is the opportunity to help patients match up the other names and faces to whom they have been exposed.

Keep in mind that the patient (usually) didn't request the consult — another doctor did. The onus is on you to develop rapport and facilitate the interview.

The following points are important to include at the beginning of the interview (though you can be flexible about the order):

- Review the patient's medical problems and progress
- State the reason for the consult
- Give an approximate idea of the length of the interview and broadly what you will be asking
- You may need to obtain permission to speak with others (family members, family doctor, community psychiatrist, etc.) in order to obtain more information
- Explain that you will have to provide a report (summary of the interview) back to the referring doctor, and you can't guarantee strict confidentiality of what the patient shares with you

In most cases, patients will speak quite readily, especially if you don't ask anything too "psychiatric" at the outset. Common approaches to focusing the interview are as follows:

- Ask what the person's emotional reaction has been to the illness
- Empathize with the degree of difficulty the person has had at work and in personal relationships
- Indicate that the referring doctor was concerned, and ask in what way the person agrees with this opinion

The priorities in conducting the consult interview are as follows:

1. Answer the consult question.

This is essential. Keep this first and foremost in mind as you go through your preparation and interview. If the need arises, refine the request according to the situation.

2. Ask about other areas that will yield information relevant to the admission or management of the medical illness.

Common areas that need exploration regardless of the consult request are: suicidal or homicidal ideation; capacity to consent to medical treatment (and in some cases capacity to manage finances); substance abuse.

3. Determine if the patient might benefit from ongoing psychiatric treatment (e.g. psychotherapy) for a condition that is not necessarily related to the medical illness.

This can be part of a psychiatric "review of symptoms" that takes place if time permits. For example, an anxiety disorder discovered while asking a set of routine screening questions could be treated with cognitive therapy while the person is still in hospital.

Asking about the presence of other disorders can detect some of the rarer (or least reported) psychiatric conditions, such as: phobic disorders, delusional disorders, and some personality disorders, etc. However, trying to fulfil this third aspect can have potential drawbacks. Eliciting information not directly related to the consult question raises the issue of confidentiality. Should all information be put in a consult note? Should the consult note be placed on the medical chart where all disciplines have access to it? Should there be a brief note for the chart and a detailed one for the private records of the consultee? There is also the etiquette factor of not "stealing" patients. While you have a responsibility to the patient, situations that fall in this area should be cleared with, and arranged through, the referring physician.

Consultation interviews tend to be short and focused. There are frequent interruptions, and often the patient cannot participate in a lengthy interview. This reinforces the need to prepare for the interview as completely as possible and to ask questions that yield the highest amount of information.

At times, you may have to reword questions because of the presence of other patients or visitors in the room. There are certain areas that may have to be omitted because of their sensitivity (e.g. childhood sexual abuse) or because they have a lesser relevance to the consultation question (for example, some aspects of the personal and family history).

You will also have to tailor the interview to suit the nature of the request. A patient you are seeing only once may require a more thorough interview than someone who will be in hospital for several weeks.

It is important to keep in mind that despite what the arrangement regarding admission appears to be at the time of the interview, this can and will change. Patients can be transferred to different hospitals, sign themselves out or be unexpectedly discharged. While there is always the opportunity to get more information in subsequent interviews, you may only be seeing the patient once, thus it is crucial to keep the consultation question in mind.

In a time-limited situation, it may be helpful to state the aim of your visit at the outset of the interview so you can redirect the patient to the salient matters if he or she heads off on a tangent. While most patients are cooperative and will speak with you readily, they do not usually know which pieces of information are essential and will need redirection at times.

Two other significant aspects of the C-L interview are:

- **Splitting**
- **The Mental Status Exam (MSE)**

Don't Split!
The process by which treatment or a "cure" comes about can vary considerably between psychiatry and medical/surgical units. Whereas psychiatric inpatients often receive direct attention daily from mental health professionals, physically ill patients are not always in need of this degree of interaction. Instead, medications and the body's ability to heal itself (time) are relied upon to a greater degree. For example, after surgery, a daily reassessment and fine-tuning of orders often provides good medical care.

When a psychiatric consultation is arranged, the patient may well have spent more time with you than he or she did with the referring doctor on that day, or in the previous few days. This, and being interested listeners, frequently puts consultants in the position of being a sounding board for patients' concerns. This occurs in three main contexts:

> • Complaints that the referring physician doesn't spend enough time with the patient, or doesn't spend as much time as you are able to
> • Comments to the effect that the physician doesn't explain procedures, discuss prognosis or tell the patient what to expect for the next step in the hospitalization
> • Telling you "secrets" that aren't to be shared with others

This process is called **splitting**, which is classified as a defense mechanism used by a person to deal with others who are regarded ambivalently. The patient may come to regard you in the "all good" part of the split because you spend more time with him or her. Alternatively, you may become the "all bad" one because your presence indicates the person has a "mental disorder." Be vigilant for signs that splitting is occurring. Use this opportunity to defend the reputation of your colleagues and do not collude with an "us vs. them" attitude. If you have genuine concerns about someone's care, speak to the consultee directly. A common intervention in these situations is to have all the members of the treatment team (attending, nurses, housestaff, etc.) meet with the patient.

The MSE

The MSE is as critical to the psychiatric interview as the physical exam is to other areas of medicine. With cognitively impaired patients, such as those with delirium, advanced dementia or severe psychosis, the MSE may be the only part of the interview that is possible to perform. The components of this exam are listed below. This mnemonic is helpful because it lists the parameters of the MSE in the order that they are often asked about and presented.

"ABC STAMP LICKER"*

Appearance
Behavior
Cooperation

Speech
Thought — **form** and **content**
Affect — visible moment-to-moment variation in
      emotion
Mood — subjective emotional tone throughout the
      interview
Perception — in all sensory modalities

Level of consciousness
Insight & Judgment
Cognitive functioning & Sensorium
      Orientation
      Memory
      Attention & Concentration
      Reading & Writing
Knowledge base
Endings — suicidal and/ or homicidal ideation
Reliability of the information supplied

*From the book:
   Brain Calipers, The Psychiatric Mental Status Exam
   David J. Robinson, M.D.
   © Rapid Psychler Press, 1997
   ISBN 0-9680324-3-5, CD-ROM 0-9682094-0-8

With time, C-L psychiatrists become very efficient interviewers and start the process of **hypothesis generation** soon after speaking to patients, and with only a limited amount of information. The consultation interview differs from a standard psychiatric interview, an emergency room interview, and a psychotherapy assessment interview.

This is one of the few times when patients who (usually) did not request to see a psychiatrist are being asked to share personal information. C-L interviews frequently involve moving to a quiet room, asking others to give you privacy, speaking to patients while they are recumbent, etc. Discussions about medical problems and hospital issues commonly precede inquiries about areas in the psychiatric realm.

A warm, empathic greeting, and thorough explanation is often required before information is gathered from the patient. The interviewer may need to work harder to gain rapport with patients in C-L interviews.

Interview Vignette

Dr. Eager: "Mr. Prazolam?"

Mr. Prazolam: "Yes."

Dr. Eager: "Good morning. I'm Dr. Eager, did Dr. Orthofreud say anything about my stopping by to speak with you?"

Mr. Prazolam: "Dr. Orthofreud. . . I haven't seen her since the operation two days ago. I'm glad you're here! I really want to get rid of this catheter. Oh, and while you're here, my usual medications haven't been given to me and I'm quite thirsty."

Dr. Eager: "Well, I'm here to help with some of those things, but I don't work on Dr. Orthofreud's team. I'm from the Psychiatry Department."

Mr. Prazolam: "That's just great. I break my hip, have an operation, lie here for two days not sleeping and now a shrink shows up. I suppose you're going to ask how I feel about that."

Dr. Eager: "How about if I explain a few things about what's happened, and then maybe you'll let me ask some questions."

Mr. Prazolam: "I'd sure like to know what's going on, but I'm not too happy about this."

Dr. Eager: "What in particular do you find upsetting?"

Mr. Prazolam: "Well, I broke my hip. I've had some pain and haven't slept well. Maybe I've been kind of nervous and edgy with the nurses. Now they send someone from your department."

Dr. Eager: "I can understand that you might be upset that no one told you I was coming to speak with you. Is there anything else about this that bothers you?"

Mr. Prazolam: "Yeah, sure. If they sent one of you people, it means everything I'm going through isn't real — it's all in my head, and now I'm cracking up. What's next? The men in white coats? A rubber room? I've seen *One Flew Over the Cuckoo's Nest.*"

Dr. Eager: "I saw the movie too. Frankly, if that was my only exposure to psychiatry, I'd be upset as well. Psychiatrists do a lot of different things, especially in general hospitals like this one."

Mr. Prazolam: "So why are you here?"

Dr. Eager: "As you mentioned a few minutes ago, I hear things haven't been going that well since the surgery. While you haven't seen Dr. Orthofreud, her team has been seeing you regularly and noticed the way things were going. They thought you seemed   anxious, and at times, depressed. Also, they asked for advice on one of your medications. So you see, they have some pretty valid reasons for asking someone to speak with you."

Mr. Prazolam: "Well, wouldn't anyone be upset with a broken hip? You don't see everyone on this ward do you?"

Dr. Eager: "No, that's true. We only see people that we're specifically asked to see. Then we provide a report back to the attending physician, which in your case is Dr. Orthofreud."

Mr. Prazolam: "So what makes me so special?"

Dr. Eager: "I had a chance to read over your chart a couple of minutes ago so I have an idea what has happened. As far as I can understand — and please correct me if I'm wrong — it seems you were confused at home, became disoriented and fell down the stairs, causing you to break your hip."

Mr. Prazolam: "That's about right."

Dr. Eager: "Well, one of the medications you take is in the Valium® family, and it can sometimes cause people to become confused. There was some concern that you had taken some extra pills, and this might have led to the confusion."

Mr. Prazolam: "Yes, I did take some extras. They stopped calming my nerves, and I took more to keep my head straight."

Dr. Eager: "Can you tell me what was going on before you increased the dosage? There's obviously some concern about you taking this medication again. Maybe another solution can be found."

Mr. Prazolam: "This goes a few months back. You see, I was traveling down a highway and I noticed a car ahead of me start to weave in the lane. It was early in the morning so I didn't think it was a drunk driver and I followed for a couple of miles in case the driver pulled over with mechanical problems. Well, the guy had been up all night and fell asleep at the wheel. The car veered off the road and hit the concrete base of an overpass. I stopped as soon as I could, but the car immediately burst into flames and there was no way of getting close to the driver."

Dr. Eager: "That's terrible. What a shock it must have been."

Mr. Prazolam: "Yeah, it was terrible, alright. Anyway they figured the guy died on impact so it wasn't like he suffered or anything. But ever since then, I've had a lot of trouble focusing on my driving, especially when I'm on my own."

Dr. Eager: "What exactly is it that you experience?"

Mr. Prazolam: "I got these sudden flashes like my life was going to end — racing heart, trouble breathing, things like that."

Dr. Eager: "What did you do after this started happening?"

Mr. Prazolam: "I fought it for a while, then I went to see my family doctor and she started me on this medication. It worked pretty well for a while, but then it didn't do anything for me."

Dr. Eager: "Was that all that happened?"

Mr. Prazolam: "No, there was more. I kept feeling guilty about the guy. Here I was watching him bob around in the lane, maybe I should have beeped my horn or tried to get him to pull over."

Dr. Eager: "So there was some lingering guilt on your part as a result of the accident. How bad did this become?"

Mr. Prazolam: "I work as a truck driver. After the pills calmed me down, I was able to drive better but I couldn't focus as well. I started taking on more and more short runs, but they don't pay as good. Some of my expenses weren't being paid and I got pretty down about it because I'm usually paid right up."

Dr. Eager: "How would you say you were different than your usual self when you were feeling down?"

Mr. Prazolam: "I pretty much had trouble sleeping and concentrating on the job."

Dr. Eager: "Anything else?"

Mr. Prazolam: "That was it mainly. I started using more of those pills because I didn't feel as bad about my problems."

Dr. Eager: "How many were you taking when your use was at its highest?"

Mr. Prazolam: "At the most, it got to twenty pills a day."

Dr. Eager: "When did the fall occur?"

Mr. Prazolam: "About four days after I starting taking that many."

Dr. Eager: "What else can you tell me about the days just before the fall?"

Mr. Prazolam: "Very little. It's really a blur to me now."

Dr. Eager: "Well, did things get so bad that you thought life wasn't worth living?"

Mr. Prazolam: "You mean like suicide? No, I didn't take them to overdose. Is that why you're here?"

Dr. Eager: "Partly for that, yes. I think you can understand how that would be something we'd ask about."

Mr. Prazolam: "Yeah, I guess so. But no, not me."

Dr. Eager: "I'm relieved to hear that, Mr. Prazolam. Another reason I'm here is to ask if you would be interested in a medication for your anxiety that didn't cause these sorts of problems, and in meeting someone on a regular basis to discuss what's happened to you? I think it would be helpful given all you've gone through."

Mr. Prazolam: "Sure. By the way, you can call me Al."

The Consult as a Commodity

Many health care professionals eschew the application of business principles to their work. Nevertheless, a "commodity" analogy is a very appropriate one for C-L psychiatry. As discussed, the interaction is far more extensive than a simple dyadic relationship between consultant and consultee.

Miller (1973) sought to define the consultation process more fully by using a **general systems model**. Guggenheim (1978), in an enjoyable and prophetic article, likened the model more to that of a marketplace where the consultation is seen as a product that must be effectively marketed.

An unfortunate reality in C-L psychiatry is that consult requests are optional for a significant percentage of patients. As discussed, process, local or even arbitrary variables are often the deciding factors as to whether referrals are made. Guggenheim aptly described this as being the major area where general systems theory fails to accurately define the consultation process:

Unfortunately, the theory as presented to date has not taken into account complexities of the general hospital as a socio-logical structure with powerful opinion-swinging constituencies that can accept or reject the consultant. It has also failed to focus on the consultant's roles as good-will ambassador and salesman (in addition to his usual roles as physician, psychiatrist, and psychotherapist).

Success in C-L psychiatry will certainly be influenced by the same factors that affect goods or services in the business world. One of the most important shifts in conceptualizing consult services in general hospitals is switching from a sales perspective ("This department has an excellent C-L service, how are you going to use it?") to a marketing perspective ("Tell us what you need from a C-L service and we will develop/ deliver it."). Unfortunately, the ability to perform a consult fulfills only part of what is required. Burket (1993) found that the features most valued by pediatricians requesting psychiatric referrals were accessibility and a timely response from consultants. Just as in business, the C-L team's image and reputation will influence referral patterns. Accordingly, there are "marketplace" aspects to consultations:

• **Advertising** e.g. letting consultees know about the progress/ improvement of patients from past referrals
• **Promotion** e.g. your presence on the medical-surgical wards or at their rounds
• **Merchandising** e.g. tailoring aspects of the consultation (notes, recommendations, disposition, etc.) to suit consultees

Because local variables (e.g. Dr. Froyd gets a lot of consults from Dr. Woods because they play golf together) so strongly influence the consultation process, it is helpful to see referring sources as customers who give us their repeat business.

References

A.S. Bagheri, L.S. Lane, F.M. Kline & D.M. Araujo
Why Physicians Fail to Tell Patients A Psychiatrist Is Coming
Psychosomatics 22(5): p. 407 — 419, 1981

R.C. Burket & J.D. Hodgin
Pediatricians' Perceptions of Child Psychiatry Consultations
Psychosomatics 34(5): p. 402 — 408, 1993

P.J. Fink
Dealing With Psychiatry's Stigma
Hospital & Community Psychiatry 37: p. 814 — 818, 1987

R. Golinger, M.L. Teitelbaum & M.F. Folstein
Clarity of Request for Consultation: Its Relationship to Psychiatric Diagnosis
Psychosomatics 26(8): p. 649 — 653, 1985

F.G. Guggenheim
A Marketplace Model of Consultation Psychiatry in the General Hospital
American Journal of Psychiatry 135(11): p. 1380 — 1383, 1978

Z.J. Lipowski
Review of Consultation Psychiatry and Psychosomatic Medicine
Psychosomatic Medicine 29: p. 153 — 171, 1967

Z. J. Lipowski
Consultation-Liaison Psychiatry: An Overview
American Journal of Psychiatry 131: p. 623 — 630, 1974

W.B. Miller
Psychiatric Consultation I: A General Systems Approach
Psychiatric Medicine 4: p. 135 — 146, 1973

S.K. Schiff & M.L. Pilot
An Approach to Psychiatric Consultation in a General Hospital
Archives of General Psychiatry 1: p. 349 — 357, 1959

Conducting Psychiatric Consultations — Explained

H. Steinberg, M. Torem & S.M. Saravary
An Analysis of Physician Resistance to Psychiatric Consultation
Archives of General Psychiatry 37: p. 1007 — 1012, 1980

T.L. Thompson II, T.N. Wise, A.B. Kelley & L.S. Mann
Improving Psychiatric Consultations to Nonpsychiatric Physicians
Psychosomatics 31(1), p. 80 — 84, 1990

J. Wallen, H.A. Pincus, H. H. Goldman & S.E. Markus
Psychiatric Consultation in Short-term General Hospitals
Archives of General Psychiatry 44:p. 163 — 168, 1987

T.N. Wise
What to Expect From a Psychiatric Consultant
Primary Care 4: p. 661— 668, 1977

T.N. Wise, L.S. Manley, H.W. Dove, E. Pluchik & K.W. Keirnan
Patients' Perceptions of Psychiatric Consultations
Comprehensive Psychiatry 26(6): p. 554 — 557, 1985

3/ Writing the Consultation Report

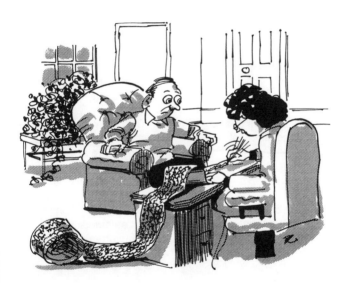

The consultation report is a unique medical document. It differs from other notes by not being written primarily for medico-legal reasons, to record progress or assist the writer's memory. The consult note serves many, and at times, contradictory functions.

In Theory ☺	In Reality ☹
The note is a doctor-to-doctor communication. . .	The consult may have been initiated by the patient, family, etc.
The note should be thorough. . .	Interest in the note is often inversely proportional to its length
Medical records should be kept confidential. . .	The note is placed on the chart for all clinical services to see — including research and insurance reviews
The note contains an outline for a treatment plan. . .	Recommendations do not automatically become orders (the patient is not under the direct care of the consultant)
The note should be an accurate record of the interview. . .	Patients can review their records at any time and may see certain aspects as pejorative (e.g. descriptions of their appearance, or when certain diagnoses are given)

Goals for the Consultation Report

- Above all else, answer the consult question
- Succinctly summarize the psychiatric problems; Popkin (1980) found that with a shorter note, there was a higher chance that drug recommendations were implemented
- Include a *Review of Symptoms* and *Mental Status Exam* to document the rationale on how you formed your diagnostic impression and treatment plan
- Outline a practical treatment plan involving biological, social, and psychological factors with appropriate investigations and short/longer term treatments
- If desired and appropriate, provide a brief, focused educational aspect to the consult (such as actual articles, references, and personal experiences)

Many clinicians take notes during the interview, especially to record the cognitive functions in the MSE. These notes are useful to refer to when composing a formal consultation report but are unlikely to be sufficient in their original form.

It is a common practice to include a handwritten note, usually from one to three pages in length, at the end of the consult. This provides immediate feedback for the consultee. Another popular practice is to speak with the referring source after the consult, often to give your opinion and present treatment options. This discussion can include the highlights of your findings, but rarely includes all the detail that would be contained in a consult note.

Depending on service requirements and the availability of clerical staff, a second dictated note is also sometimes provided. This note is usually more detailed, and can serve as a record for findings or impressions that are tactfully left off the chart on the medical floor. Notes of this type are especially helpful for patients:

- With complicated histories
- With sensitive historical information
- Who are likely to require repeat consultations

Despite the many advantages of speaking with referring sources both before and after the consult, your note may be the only contact they have with the C-L Service. If your sole interaction with others is going to take place via the chart, then your initial note becomes the calling card which sets the stage for the nature and quality of further exchanges. Those reading the chart will attest to your brilliance (or lack of it) based on your ability to compose a crisp, accurate, and useful note. For this reason, it is useful to consider your note as being an ambassador to the foreign territory of medical-surgical units. This concept will be expanded further in outlining the sections generally included in a consult note.

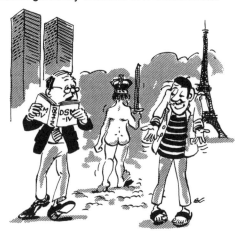

Don't just dispatch a Page, send an Ambassador!

The Well-Composed Ambassador

Here are the key elements for composing your ambassador:

A Sense of Entitlement
The consultation note requires a title. Some departments have preprinted forms with a prominent heading, as well as check boxes for other relevant information. Most hospitals have generic consult forms for all services. These frequently come assembled as carbonless copies so that the referring physician, medical records, and the consultant can all have a copy. Lastly, if no forms are available, the note can be written on hospital paper and placed in the "Consultations" or "Progress" section of the chart.

A Proper Introduction
A one or two sentence "identifying statement" usually starts off the formal note. These parameters are often relevant to the prognosis and treatment planning, and are important to include at the outset. However, the referring source already knows this, so be brief. It is vital to include the date of the interview, often with the time (and time period) the person was seen. Some clinicians routinely list the sources of information used in the consult (e.g. patient, family, general practitioner, chart, etc.). Others only include this information if the assessment is incomplete, or if the patient was not the primary source of data. The length of stay in hospital prior to the consult can also be included.

A Well-Informed Opening
After the identifying information, it is common to include a one or two sentence summary of the patient's:

- Medical or surgical problem/ reason for admission
- Course and severity
- Recent or proposed procedures

Again, this information is known to the referring source. Brevity is advisable because you haven't as yet added anything new — so include only what is relevant to the immediate problem.

A Clear Sense of Purpose
The next section states the reason for the referral and possibly the consultee's expectations. This can consist of simply restating the request, rewording it into a more typical request, or, in cases where the reason wasn't explicitly stated, describing what to you seems to be the most appropriate reason for the referral. As stated previously, the reason for referral is often omitted from the consult request, but is important to include in a formal note.

This is also not the time or place to involve sarcasm or highlighting the lack of psychological mindedness of some of our colleagues. Requests such as the following should be reworded:

- "Please stop this patient's hallucinations"
- "Assess and change the patient's personality"
- "Tell the patient to be nicer to the nursing staff"
- "Advise on proper anticonfusional medication"

The reason for referral becomes the focus of the consult. Along with an understanding of the consultee's expectations, this forms the basis of your recommended treatment plan, and in a sense forms the "contract" for the consult.

A Thorough Grounding in Current Events
The next section, the **History of Presenting Illness (HPI)**, details the events leading up to the consult request. This section starts at the point where the patient was last well (or was last his or her "usual self") and details the medical, psychiatric, and interpersonal factors necessary to understand how

the person came to be in the current situation at the time the consult was requested.

This section diverges from the medical/surgical style and takes on a distinctly psychiatric flavor. Symptoms are presented which are relevant to the medical problem and which lead to a psychiatric diagnosis. All aspects which are relevant to the patient's current difficulties are listed here. These can include factors such as medications, family, and job stresses, substance abuse, etc. Significant negative findings are also listed in this section.

Understanding Past as Prologue
The **psychiatric history** is often the next section included which chronicles the following information:

- Previous admissions
- Other contact with mental health professionals
- Type, duration, and response to psychotherapy
- Treatment with medications and outcome
- Substance abuse that is in remission or considered not contributing to the current difficulties

For the sake of brevity, this section can also be used for recording information that might be placed in the Personal/ Social and Family History in a full psychiatric history. Other significant aspects that can be recorded in this section are:

- Past responses to stressful events/ losses
- Characteristic coping patterns (personality style)
- Anniversary dates of significant losses
- Relatives affected by psychiatric conditions

The Directive of the "Mental State"
The **MSE** is an essential area of evaluation in consultation psychiatry. This structured set of inquiries assesses cogni-

tive functions and the symptoms of psychiatric illness not covered elsewhere in the interview. Documenting the MSE is like recording the "objective" part of the **Subjective/ Objective/ Assessment/ Plan (S.O.A.P.)** approach. Positive findings from the MSE illustrate how psychiatric diagnoses and recommendations are based on detailed, structured inquiries.

The MSE has a significant likelihood of being abnormal because of the higher prevalence of cognitive impairment (delirium, dementia, etc.) in medically ill patients with psychiatric problems. Remember that the MSE is a snapshot of a person's mental functioning — it can and will vary with time. The MSE can be supplemented with other cognitive screening tests like the **Mini-Mental State Exam (MMSE)** and clock drawing.

Seeing Between The Lines
A **Review of Symptoms (ROS)** is frequently included in consultation notes. For many patients who are referred, the consult will be their only contact with a psychiatrist. Exploring other diagnostic possibilities that are related to the core symptoms is a very worthwhile exercise because:

> • It helps detect occult psychiatric illnesses
> • It establishes you as a thorough consultant, and the referring source will request more consults

While the questions in this area can take a few minutes to ask, the documentation can be brief. You can list the individual psychiatric conditions screened for as being not present, or list the overall categories. For example:

> • "Negative screen for psychotic, anxiety and somatoform disorders"
> • "Screened for anxiety disorders other than Panic Disorder — OCD, PTSD, Phobias (including Agoraphobia) & GAD not present"

A Unifying Stance

An **impression**, **summary** or **formulation** follows next. Many times this and the proposed treatment plan will be all that the primary physician reads. This section is usually a paragraph in length and starts with significant identifying factors, the medical problem, and the course/ severity of that illness.

Then, the positive psychiatric symptoms are highlighted and correlated into a **provisional**, **preferred** or **working diagnosis**. A **differential diagnosis** is also included, and may be emphasized in cases with higher degrees of complexity. Detailing the process of collecting information from the patient (and other sources), identifying symptoms, and then distilling them into a diagnostic formulation makes your rationale for suggesting investigations and treatments (both biological and psychosocial) clear to the referring source, and increases the likelihood of their implementation.

Treatment Planning & Recommendations

If the previous sections of the consult note answer the question, *"What is going on with this patient? "* then the treatment plan answers the question, *"What do we do about it? "* Primary physicians have a varying interest in your ability to conduct an interview and arrive at an elegant diagnostic formulation, but there will be universal interest in your expertise in directly helping to manage their patients. Your treatment plan is the most important part of the consult and may be the only part that gets read. Generally, your outline becomes a list of suggestions for the referring team who may or may not agree with your ideas. The degree to which consultees follow recommendations has been termed **concordance**, and is discussed in a separate chapter.

Following a biopsychosocial outline, one approach is to consider which investigations are called for, and then which short and longer-term treatments will benefit the patient. An outline of the most common parameters in these areas appears in the next section.

Investigations are most frequently ordered to help distinguish disorders that have a demonstrable physiologic basis. Such disorders are still frequently called "organic," to draw a distinction from causes deemed to be entirely psychiatric or "functional" illnesses (sometimes still called "supratentorial"). The DSM-IV terminology for this is **Mental Disorder Due to a General Medical Condition**. For example, someone who clearly develops a major depressive episode due to Cushing's Disease would be diagnosed in the following manner:

> *Axis I*   Mood Disorder due to Cushing's Disease, with Depressive Features
> *Axis III* Cushing's Disease

Where the etiology is less clearly related, the diagnosis would be recorded as:

> *Axis I*   Major Depressive Disorder
> *Axis III* Cushing's Disease

Biopsychosocial Management Plan

> • **Is admission to hospital necessary?**
>
> • **Does the patient require an involuntary admission?**

Investigations

Biological
- Admission physical exam
- Diagnostic tests:
    - *Routine*: hematologic and clinical chemistry admission/ screening bloodwork

> *Toxicology*: serum medication levels; urine screen for substances of abuse
> *Special assays*

- Diagnostic investigations: CXR, EKG
- Neuroimaging: CT, MRI scans
- EEG
- Consultations to other medical/surgical specialties
- Special tests:
  > *hypothalamic/ pituitary/ adrenal axis testing (DST, TRH stimulation test, GH response)*
  > *sleep studies*
  > *other*

Social

- Collateral history:
  > *friends and family members*
  > *primary care physician*
  > *community psychiatrist*
  > *other clinics, programs or hospitals*
- Activities of Daily Living (**ADL**) and Instrumental Activities of Daily Living (**IADL**) assessment
- Referral to members of multidisciplinary team
  > *Social Worker*
  > *Occupational Therapist, Physiotherapist*
  > *Dietician*
  > *Clergy*
  > *Nurse Clinician*

Psychological

- Personality and Intelligence tests
- Cognitive screening tests (e.g. Mini-Mental State Exam, Clock Drawing, etc.)
- Neuropsychological test batteries
- Structured interviews/ diagnostic testing

Treatment — Short Term

Biological
- Psychopharmacology
  - *antidepressants*
  - *antiparkinsonian agents*
  - *antipsychotics*
  - *anxiolytics*
  - *mood stabilizers*
  - *psychostimulants*
  - *sedative/ hypnotics*
  - *other*
- ECT
- Other psychiatric treatments
- Somatic illnesses
  - *medications*
  - *physical treatments*
- Detoxification from medications or substances
- Environmental
  - *level of observation*
  - *passes*
  - *attire (pajamas or street clothes)*
  - *seclusion rooms*
  - *mechanical restraints*
  - *objects to assist with reorientation*

Social
- Social services
  - *assistance with housing, finances, etc.*
- Education and focus/ support groups
- Occupational Therapy
- Family meetings
- Administrative
  - *voluntary/ involuntary status*
  - *rights/ legal advice*
  - *duty to warn/ duty to protect others*

treatment contracts
informing work/ school of absence
substitute consent if deemed incapable

Psychological
- Advice/ Reality Therapy
- Behavior Therapy/ Modification
- Cognitive Therapy
- Group Therapy
- Milieu Therapy
- Recreation Therapy
- Stress Management/ Coping Skills
- Other therapies with a shorter-term focus

Treatment — Longer Term

Biological
- Reduction/ optimization of dosage
- Depot antipsychotic medications
- Monitoring vulnerable organ systems
- Serum level monitoring
- Adjunct/ augmentation/ combination treatments
- Factors reducing the efficacy of medication
    nicotine
    caffeine
    liver enzyme inducers
    others
- Health teaching and lifestyle changes

Social
- Vocational rehabilitation
- Religious guidance
- Community supports and organizations
- Discharge planning
    transfer to another facility
    case manager, general practitioner

Psychological
- Psychotherapy
  - *continuation of inpatient therapy*
  - *arrange outpatient treatment*
- Match various types of therapies to needs and attainable goals for the patient
- Types of therapies listed on next page

The Biopsychosocial Grid *

	Biological	Psychological	Social
Investigations	A	B	B
Short-Term Treatment	C	E	F
Longer-Term Treatment	D	E	F

* the letters refer to the sections on the following pages (starting on p.68) where these topics are discussed in detail

Medical Differential Diagnosis

"MASTER THIS SCID"*

Metabolic
Autoimmune
Septic/ Infectious
Traumatic
Endocrine
Renal

> SCID stands for the Structured Clinical Interview for the DSM-IV

Toxic
Hematologic/Circulatory
Idiopathic
Structural

Somatoform (Psychiatric)
Congenital
Iatrogenic
Degenerative

Treatment Modalities

"ABCDEFGHIJKLM"*

Addiction
Behavioral
Cognitive
Drug (medications)
ECT (electroconvulsive therapy)
Family Therapy
Group Therapy
Hospitalization (partial, day or inpatient)
Insight-Oriented (psychoanalysis, psychodynamic
 psychotherapy)
Job (vocational rehabilitation)
Knowledge (patient and family education)
Leisure (art therapy, music therapy, crafts groups,
 etc.)
Marital and relationship counseling

From the book:
Psychiatric Mnemonics & Clinical Guides, 2nd Edition
David J. Robinson, M.D.
Rapid Psychler Press
ISBN 0-9682094-1-6

A/ Biological Investigations

Recommending biological investigations can at times be a delicate issue. Most referrals will come to you from experts in physical medicine who will at least have initiated investigations (being "worked-up"), if not having already ordered thorough testing for their patients. With the costs of medical care escalating, many physicians are being conservative in which tests are ordered (i.e. serum levels of ozone, porcelain and marmalade are no longer routine). For this reason, certain investigations may have been considered and postponed pending clinical necessity (i.e. waiting for more common tests to be reported as within normal limits (**WNL**) before investigating less common possibilities).

Your suggestions may not be implemented because they are thought to be a low-yield proposition. Referring physicians generally do not look for psychiatric consults to direct them to order more investigations, since this is their area of expertise. Keep in mind that requesting consultations can be difficult for physicians because, in asking for assistance, it is a reminder that they are not "all capable and all knowing." While many physicians accept that psychiatry is different enough from physical medicine that they will readily request your help, recommendations for biochemical or hematologic tests may be misconstrued to mean that you don't feel they are demonstrating capable medical skills.

Explaining the clinical necessity of your ideas rather than exchanging notes in the chart goes a long way to insuring that they will be carried out. If you have a high index of suspicion, work collaboratively with the referring team by telling them your concerns and allowing them to direct the investigations.

The tests most likely to be accepted are those that fall under the domain of psychiatry. For example, the ordering of lithium, carbamazepine or valproate levels is often not done routinely and will be relevant to the consult. Additionally, testing of organ systems affected by such medications (e.g. liver function tests, blood cell counts, thyroid function) is more likely to be carried out.

Alternatively, not every member of every team considers the myriad of psychological consequences that can be caused or maintained by physical illnesses.

There are certain situations that may require you to order routine tests or to be more assertive in seeing that your suggestions are carried out:

Beginning of Rotations or Academic Years.

Temporary Lack of Supervision for a Medical Team.
Medical students, clinical clerks, residents, fellows, and students in other clinical programs work in hospitals because an apprenticeship is required in addition to classroom material. No one learns to swim by reading a book, and this is reflected in the often heard statement, "the last time I saw a textbook case was in a textbook."

Referral Early in the Admission.
Some consults are requested at the outset of an admission and not all the tests will have been ordered prior to your visit. While it is always a benefit to being called earlier than later, you may need to postpone your investigations or recommendations pending the test results.

In the vast majority of cases, adequate testing will have been ordered. However, you may find that not all results have been reported and you can call the lab for the values.

You may infrequently discover a medical disorder that hasn't yet been detected (e.g. Wilson's Disease, lead poisoning, hypothyroidism). In general, consultees appear more interested in management recommendations than in investigations (Popkin, 1983). However, Popkin (1982) also found that consultees have an inclination to prematurely terminate the work-up of patients with psychiatric symptoms.

Important Organic Considerations

"TIME WON'T PASS"

Trauma — particularly head injuries and intracranial bleeding
Infections — especially of the CNS
Multiple sclerosis
Epilepsy

Wilson's Disease — an inherited defect in copper metabolism
Obstruction of CSF — Normal Pressure Hydrocephalus (NPH)
Nutritional — e.g. vitamin deficiencies, protein-deficient diets
Toxic — ingestion of medication, heavy metals, chemicals, etc.

Porphyria, **P**heochromocytoma
Axis of hypothalamus-pituitary-thyroid-adrenal glands
Space-Occupying Lesions
Substances — abuse, tolerance, intoxication and withdrawal states

Hall (1980) investigated the prevalence of medical illnesses that caused or exacerbated psychiatric symptoms (left column below). The right column lists the investigations useful in detecting these illnesses. These investigations are ranked by Hall from most to least useful:

Illnesses		Investigations
• Endocrine	43%	• Blood chemistry — 34 panel
• CNS	19%	• Complete physical exam
• Hematologic	19%	• History
• Cardiovascular	9%	• Complete blood count
• Gastrointestinal	6%	• Blood chemistry — 12 panel
• Genitourinary	2%	• Sleep-deprived EEG
• Musculoskeletal	2%	• ECG
		• Routine urinalysis
		• Cursory physical exam
		• Complete neurological exam

B/ Social & Psychological Investigations

These investigations are far less likely to rankle consultees. Such investigations traditionally fall under the rubric of the behavioral sciences and are not typically assessments that the referring team would or could carry out without your help. In the interest of efficiency, check to see if anyone from the referring team has undertaken any of the following actions:

- Requested old charts
- Contacted the family doctor
- Arranged a family meeting

Usually, you will be required to speak with the collateral sources of information that are more socially/ psychologically oriented. This typically involves contacting: community agencies, schools or places of employment.

On occasion, specialized neuropsychological testing will be necessary (the deficits to be further explored will of course be detected in your initial MSE). The most common mental functions assessed are: memory; reasoning and problem solving; perceptual performance; intelligence; language; motor skills; orientation, attention & concentration. Some of the tests most frequently ordered to assess mental functions are:

- Luria-Nebraska Neuropsychologic Battery
- Halsted-Reitan Battery
- Wisconsin Card Sorting Test
- Wechsler Adult Intelligence Scale — Revised (WAIS-R)
- **ADLs & IADLs**

Other psychological testing may be needed to assess personality. These are divided into **objective tests** (e.g. MMPI) and **projective tests** (e.g. Rorschach, Thematic Apperception Test, etc.). In order to more fully document your diagnoses, there are various Structured Clinical Diagnostic Assessments.

C/ Short-Term Biological (Psychopharmacological) Treatments

Having a thorough knowledge of the indications, side-effects, and contraindications of both psychiatric and non-psychiatric medications is a necessity in C-L psychiatry. Psychiatric drugs can cause a wide variety of medical complications (e.g. orthostatic hypotension, hepatotoxicity, galactorrhea/amenorrhea, agranulocytosis, etc.). Similarly, drugs for medical conditions can cause a plethora of psychological reactions (mania, depression, psychosis, anxiety, dissociation, sleep disorders, personality changes, etc.). While the list of possible reactions is quite extensive, it is imperative to keep the more common sequelae in mind. An important clinical pearl in this regard is to always keep an index of suspicion and look for factors that may have precipitated the patient's difficulties.

Because of the decreasing length of inpatient stays, medications are a very important part of a consultant's armamentarium. Many agents will work in a span of hours to days (e.g. benzodiazepines, antipsychotics). Because some have a longer period to onset (e.g. mood stabilizers, antidepressants), it is important to get such medications started as soon as possible.

A question to always consider is, "At this time, what is/are the right psychiatric medication(s) for a patient with these physical illnesses?" Dealing with inpatients has advantages in the area of psychopharmacology:

- Compliance is very good (but not 100%)
- A variety of routes of administration are possible (oral, intravenous, sublingual, rectal, intramuscular, transdermal)
- You have the chance to monitor daily progress
- There are many caregivers to assess side effects
- Serious reactions/side effects can be dealt with quickly

On the other hand, inpatient prescribing does have special concerns. Patients may be cognitively impaired and not be able to give informed consent. There may be factors related to hospitalization (noisy rooms, bad food) that get reported as side effects (poor sleep and decreased appetite, respectively). While a comprehensive discussion of C-L psychopharmacology is beyond the scope of this book, a list of some of the more relevant clinical points follows for the major groups of medication.

Antipsychotics
• Usually safe to give, but the traditional agents have effects on most neurotransmitter systems, so side-effects abound
• Many medical/surgical staff have not seen, or will be slower to recognize **neuroleptic malignant syndrome**, **dystonic reactions**, **akathisia** and **pseudoparkinsonism**
• Newer antipsychotics are not available in parenteral forms

Anticholinergic Agents
• Staff may need instruction on what to look for and how to give these medications (i.e., IM injection in severe cases)
• Anticholinergic effects are additive to the effects of the antipsychotics, which can lead to **anticholingeric toxicity**
• Akathisia does not respond to this group of medications

Antidepressants
• While frequently prescribed, the delay in onset of action requires use after discharge, so you need to involve the G.P.
• Older agents have more side effects and induce more manic episodes in patients with Bipolar Mood Disorder; these drugs have many clinical uses that newer agents (currently) don't
• Newer antidepressants are better tolerated and much safer when taken in overdose, but are more expensive and may be stigmatized because of the popularity of Prozac®

Mood Stabilizers
• All require blood levels and organ system monitoring
• May affect the efficacy of other medications (e.g. hepatic metabolism induction by carbamazepine)
• There is a delayed action for mood symptom control
• Anticonvulsants have a significant risk of teratogenesis
• Lithium needs to be given cautiously to patients who are not adequately hydrated (e.g. post-op, n.p.o.); levels should be drawn 12h after the last dose

Antianxiety Agents

• Benzodiazepines are the most commonly prescribed drugs in this category, but others can be used (e.g. buspirone, propranolol, some tricyclic antidepressants, hydroxyzine, etc.)
• The longer the half-life of the medication, the more it will affect daytime alertness (i.e. "a hangover" effect); on the other hand, shorter acting compounds have a higher abuse potential due to rebound anxiety
• Lorazepam, oxazepam and temazepam are rapidly metabolized by direct conjugation and do not have active metabolites — these are important considerations in patients with liver disease (e.g. due to alcohol dependence)

Hypnotics

• Again, benzodiazepines are popular but can lead to dependence if given for a period longer than two weeks
• REM cycles are affected by benzodiazepines
• Other medications are available (e.g. chloral hydrate, zolpidem, zopiclone)
• Discussing sleep hygiene with patients may reduce or remove the need for medications; many people sleep poorly in hospital due to the noise, strange bed, roommates, etc.

Stimulants

• May need to be given to those who have treatment-resistant depression
• Patients who are receiving palliative care and have become depressed may be candidates due to the speed of onset and efficacy of these medications in elevating mood

General Considerations

• Because many referring physicians treat illnesses with medications, they often expect you to prescribe *something*
• Because patients receive a number of medications in hospital, be vigilant for potential interactions
• You are the primary source of information for psychotropic

medications (and for obtaining consent), a few moments spent explaining such matters can be very helpful

D/ Longer-Term Medication Considerations

Outlining longer-term medication considerations is usually not done in the initial consult note. These factors become relevant as the admission progresses and when the patient's response to your original recommendations is known.

If you are going to see the person once or only for a short time, it is helpful to include a management outline. For example, if a patient is being started on lithium, you might include the following helpful points in your note:

- Reminders about measuring drug levels and when to do so (e.g. 4 — 7 days after a dosage change)
- The serum range for acute treatment
- Lab indices to monitor (e.g. leukocytosis)

Other general considerations include:

- If the medication should be continued upon discharge
- If you will be following the patient or will contact the G.P. to offer advice on the long term use
- If alternate preparations are available or should be considered (e.g. suspensions instead of pills, depot forms of neuroleptics, sustained-release tablets) and possible dosing arrangements (e.g. once daily, bid, tid, etc.)

E/ Psychological and Psychotherapeutic Treatments

While referring teams may modify your suggested biological investigations and treatments, there is usually little objection to your recommending and implementing a form of psycho-therapy with patients. As long as your sessions don't unduly upset patients or interfere with other treatments, consultees are almost always grateful that you will share your time and expertise.

The range of treatments available is impressive and expand-ing. Most of the letters in the **"ABCDEFGHIJKLM"** mnemonic (p. 67) are forms of psychotherapy. However, not all of these modalities will be available or advisable for inpatients.

The approaches most applicable to C-L psychiatry are often:

- Brief
- Reality-based
- Solution-focused
- Cognitive or educational in nature

It is usually sufficient to record in the recommendation sec-tion that ongoing psychotherapy is indicated, and that either you will be doing it, or you will speak with the person who will be doing it. You can mention the type of therapy involved and briefly state the goals that are appropriate for this interven-tion. This is especially important if the patient is engaging in behavior that is problematic for the primary physician. Here, "consultation" psychiatry provides psychotherapy for the pa-tient while "liaison" psychiatry also helps the referring team. Personality disordered patients can, through the use of un-conscious ego defense mechanisms, elicit strong responses from referring teams. For example, **projection** may engen-der hostile responses towards patients, while **splitting** may cause some consultees to behave seductively.

F/ Social Treatments

Social treatments focus on assisting patients with working and

living arrangements. For example, patients who have had ac-
cidents or who have chronic psychiatric illnesses may need
vocational rehabilitation during or after hospital stays. Some
patients will require help in finding shelters or group homes.
While there are usually social workers or other staff to assist
with these matters, keeping abreast of community agencies
and supports is important. Often there are directories available listing various resources. Social treatments can also involve linking patients with local or national self-help groups.
A list of psychosocial articles is provided in McCartney (1985).

Documenting the Consultation

The consultation note has to include a number of essential
pieces of information for academic, financial, research and
clinical reasons, yet be brief enough to be useful to consultees.
Recently, two articles have been written that provide further
guidance regarding consult notes. The sample C-L note provided in this chapter contains the recommendations set out
by Bronheim (1998) in the APM Practice Guidelines, though
three points bear emphasis: avoid using acronyms and jar-
gon, remember that records are available to third parties, and
consult notes must be signed. Worley et al (1998) provide a
structured C-L Form that complies with **Health Care Financ-
ing Administration (HCFA)** and **American Medical Association (AMA) Guidelines**. The authors warn that financial
penalties can result if the documentation cannot justify the
services that have been billed.

Sample Consultation Notes
The next section contains three medical notes:
- A medical admission note outlining the physical
aspects of a patient's illness
- An "overly psychiatric" consultation note which
provides considerable psychosocial detail
- A balanced psychiatric consultation note

> **MEDICAL ADMISSION NOTE**
> by Dr. Billy Rubin
> Dept. of Medicine PGY-2
> May 5th
> Information obtained from interview & old chart.

ID: Mr A is a 32-year-old male teacher.

RFA: Exacerbation of ulcerative colitis (UC).

HPI: Patient has had UC since age 27. Flare-ups in the past have responded well to steroid enemas and oral sulfasalazine. Had 1 bowel movement (BM) per day and no abdominal pain until 3 weeks ago. At this point, he started to have 3 — 5 BMs per day with occasional diarrhea. In the last three days he's had a diminished appetite, abdominal pain, bloody diarrhea, and chills. Mr. A reports a 5 kg/11lb. weight loss over the 3 weeks (he wasn't trying to lose weight). Vomiting intermittently now for four days. Canker sores (aphthous ulcers) on inside of lips and cheek. Pain is crampy in nature and occurs over the lower abdomen — this improves with BMs.

Denies having any arthralgias, eye problems, liver involvement or skin problems. No recent travel or unusual foods. Very stressed at work lately.

HPH: UC (5 years ago); Gastroesophageal reflux (10 years)
Benign familial tremor
Sigmoid polypectomy (1 year ago — benign)

Meds: sulfasalazine 2 g p.o. daily
loperamide 2 mg caps p.o. prn
codeine phosphate 30 mg p.o. qid

Allergies: Environmental (ragweed and pollen); none to drugs

Personal: Home-room teacher for grade 6. Never married, lives with parents. Bachelor's degree in Arts, then attended Teacher's College. His alcohol intake is minimal and he doesn't imbibe during flare-ups. Last drink was 4 weeks ago. Non-smoker, doesn't use recreational drugs.

Family: Parents and 1 younger sister all alive — none have UC. Family history of heart disease, but no known incidence of cancer (esp. bowel). Parents have had screening colonoscopies which have been normal.

Physical Exam:
Alert, oriented, and stable. Looks pale. Seems anxious and upset at times.

Vitals: BP 130/80, HR 80 and regular, RR 14, T = 38 C

HEENT: pupils equal and reactive to light; no papilledema; full extra-ocular movements; ears clear; several aphthous ulcers; mucous membranes dry

Chest: clear to IPPA, no wheezes or crackles

CVS: $S_1 S_2$ — regular rhythm, systolic ejection murmur 2/6, no elevation in JVP, peripheral pulses palpable

Abdomen: no scars or asymmetry; LKKS not palpable; no masses, bowel sounds present; DRE deferred until settled

Neuro/ MSK: CN 2 — 12 intact; no sensory deficits, DTRs are normal; no Babinski; gait is normal; cerebellar testing is WNL

Labs: Sodium — 135, Chloride — 98, Potassium — 3.5
Bicarb — 30, Urea — 3.6, Creatinine — 60
Blood Counts: Hb — 120, WBC — 10.5, Platelets — 356
ESR 80, INR 1.2, PTT 26

LFTs, RFTs, calcium, magnesium, phosphate, albumin pending

Stool C & S, blood C & S to be taken on arrival to floor

Impression: 32-year-old man with history of UC for 7 years. Has had episodic flare-ups over this time. Well until 3 weeks ago when he developed increased frequency of BMs with occasional diarrhea. Now acutely ill for 3 — 4 days with abdominal pain, blood in diarrhea and chills — all consistent with another flare-up. Oral intake is poor due to aphthous ulcers and vomiting which has led to an 11 lb. weight loss and dehydration at present. No involvement of joints, eyes, skin or liver/biliary tract at present. Compliance with medication is good.

Pt. anxious and upset during interview and examination — feels stressed at work.

Plan:
- Admit to medical team
- Rehydrate and give IV corticosteroids
- Monitor hemoglobin daily
- Arrange flexible sigmoidoscopy/colonoscopy
- Consult General Surgery and Psychiatry

PSYCHIATRIC CONSULTATION NOTE
by Dr. S. Froyd
Attending, Dept. of Psychoanalysis
May 6th 9:00 a.m.
Information obtained from patient interview

Mr. A is a 32-year-old, single, male, public school teacher who was referred for psychiatric consultation during an admission for exacerbation of ulcerative colitis. Mr. A's internist explained that he complained of depressive and anxious symptoms which he felt were related to stress at work. Mr. A's job has become more demanding as his class size increased and students with disturbed behavior and borderline normal intelligence have been included in the regular classes. Mr. A struggles to control the class' behavior and to maintain reasonable academic standards under these difficult conditions. This is a special challenge for Mr. A who tends to have high standards for himself and who is not comfortable with situations which he feels he can't control. The recent exacerbation of ulcerative colitis appears to be associated with Mr. A's feeling that he did not have his principal's support. Mr. A appears highly motivated to get the principal's approval by controlling the class' behavior and successfully completing the academic program. This has been difficult because of the disruptive behavior of these students, whom the principal will not suspend for more than three days. Mr. A appears to struggle between his wish to please the principal and his increasing resentment at the principal for not helping him deal with the situation. His anxiety increases whenever he becomes aware of his anger at the principal.

Mr. A's parents were blue collar workers who had high expectations of him. He has a younger sister who was expected to complete high school, get married, and raise a family which she did. Mr. A's father, a retired factory worker, wanted him to succeed in a profession which his father felt would bring prestige to the family and justify the sacrifices in putting Mr. A through university. Mr. A described his father as strict, demanding, and quite involved. Mr. A's father used to be pleased when Mr. A got high marks, but would express dissatisfaction at anything less than honors, and expected Mr. A to have a part-time job during high school to help pay for his university education. Mr. A felt all of this to be a considerable demand although he was anxious to please his father. He described his mother in generally positive terms as being less demanding than his father and reasonably affectionate. However, she worked at night and was available only on weekends and holidays.

Mr. A dated a number of women since leaving university, but hasn't had a relationship last for more than 12 months. He feels that women find him rather fussy and inflexible. A couple of them have indicated that they felt that he was not ready to leave his parents and make a commitment to marriage. The closest relationship he's had was with a woman he dated for 10 months at the age of 27. In spite of some ambivalence on his part, he was prepared to marry her when she unexpectedly broke off their relationship, complaining that he was still too attached to his parents.

Mr. A has always lived with his parents except for one year when he attended university in another city. This was a difficult year for him as he did not make many friends while away. He kept in almost constant telephone contact with his parents and frequently flew back for weekend visits and all holidays. Mr. A appears to have internalized his father's demanding attitude towards him, with the result that he has quite a demanding attitude towards himself. He appears to project his internal image of his father onto his principal, wishing to please the principal under circumstances which seem to be as demanding as those that he grew up with. He appears to deal with his resentment towards the principal with a reaction formation and instead, tries to please the principal. This resentment is likely amplified by his repressed resentment towards his father who the principal appears to represent for Mr. A.

Mr. A appears to have had some difficulty in separating from his parents and establishing close adult relationships. In particular, he has had difficulty in developing his own standards and ideals, and instead appears to have persisted in attempting to fulfill his father's standards in order to get his father's approval. This may be understood on the basis of his father's withholding approval unless Mr. A functioned at a very high level, on the many demands Mr. A's father made of him, and on his mother's relative unavailability. The onset and exacerbation of episodes of colitis appears related to frustrations and losses in relationships which Mr. A has not felt able to control. These include the breakup of his relationship with his girlfriend and the present difficulty with his principal, with whom he is frustrated but cannot express his anger, as he wants to please him. This is likely a repetition of the pattern he experienced over the years with his father. His mother's unavailability has likely made him more vulnerable to separation.

Diagnostic Impression: Adjustment Disorder with Mixed Emotional Features; Psychological Factors Affecting Medical Disorders; Personality Disorder with Obsessive-Compulsive and Dependent traits.

Plan: Mr. A's symptoms do not appear to warrant the prescription of a psychoactive medication. This consultant will interview him on a regular basis while he is in hospital in an attempt to establish a psychotherapeutic relationship. If Mr. A is amenable, the consultant will arrange to meet with him on a thrice-weekly basis for 50 minutes in order to begin a supportive psychotherapy in which Mr. A can explore the difficulties he is having with his principal and how these difficulties may relate to the exacerbation of his colitis. Depending on the outcome, a more ambitious psychodynamic therapy may be attempted.

PSYCHIATRIC CONSULTATION NOTE
by Dr. B. Eager, Pager 0968/Ext. 2094
PGY-3, Consultation Psychiatry Service
May 6th 2:30 — 4:30 p.m.
Information obtained from patient interview and
hospital chart
Consult requested by: Dr. G.I. Joe

I.D. Mr. A is a 32-year-old, white, single, male public school teacher currently living with his parents.

Reason for Admission Mr. A was admitted May 5th due to a flare-up of ulcerative colitis (UC) during which he became increasingly ill over a 3 week period. He was diagnosed with UC 7 years ago and has required 4 inpatient stays in this time period.

Reason for Referral Evaluation of depressive and anxious symptoms; provide continuing care while in hospital; advise on suitability of outpatient follow-up. Referral received May 6th.

History of Present Illness Mr. A was last well about 3 weeks ago. At that time, he started to experience a change in bowel habits which intensified into a systemic resurgence of his illness. He was dehydrated on admission and has a sigmoidoscopy booked for later today.

His illness has taken a toll on him emotionally, and he was noted to be "anxious and upset" during the admission interview and physical. Mr. A is currently the homeroom teacher for a Grade 6 class. He devotes a considerable amount of his time preparing lessons that "meet the letter" of the education objectives. Since the holidays, his class size has increased because several families relocated near his school. A special education teacher left and students with borderline normal intelligence were also added to his class. The increased number of students, and in particular those requiring extra attention, have disrupted his usual careful planning. Mr. A likes to have the full attention of the class, and is aware that control issues are important to him. About the time of the onset of his symptoms, two boys released a handful of insects in the class, which disrupted the entire afternoon and required a pest control company to be involved. The students were suspended by the principal for three days which is far less than the two weeks Mr. A had requested. Mr. A has worked diligently to impress the principal, and has distinguished himself. This has been the only disagreement so far.

Evaluation of depressive symptoms is as follows:

• **Sleep** — has had trouble with initial insomnia for 3 weeks, no early morning awakening, no sedative medications
• **Appetite** — diminished with flare-up, has lost 11 lbs. in 3 weeks (not desired); usually a picky eater (avoids dairy products)
• **Mood** — describes it as down persistently for 3 days; gives himself a score of 3/10 and is usually a 7 or 8
• **Interest** — able to stay up with demands of school; reads newspapers and novels; less enthusiastic this week only
• **Concentration** — unimpaired; able to recall 3/3 objects, serial 7's all correct, spelled "WORLD" backwards properly
• **Guilt/worthlessness** — describes these as continual issues for him, but no worse at this time
• **Psychomotor changes** — not observable during the interview
• **Energy** — plays squash twice-weekly; hasn't played this week due to physical condition, but otherwise energy level described as normal
• **Suicide/ Homicide** — no thoughts of harm to self or others; no past attempts to harm himself

Evaluation of anxiety symptoms is as follows:

• Anxiety is episodic, and almost always clearly related to identifiable factors; in this situation, he is concerned about his performance as a teacher and the outcome of this flare-up (e.g. will he need surgery?)
• His feelings of anxiousness last for up to 6 weeks, but vary according to the cycles of exams and teacher evaluations
• Doesn't describe discrete obsessions or compulsions, but has a pervasive drive to achieve high standards in all facets of his life
• No discrete panic attacks or life-threatening experiences
• Not afraid to go places where help/escape not easily arranged
• Not solely concerned with humiliation or embarrassment
• His fear is not cued by certain objects or situations

Review of Symptoms   No complaints or observations consistent with psychotic disorders, bipolar mood disorder, hypochondriasis, eating disorders or substance abuse/dependence.

Psychiatric History   No psychiatric admissions. He saw a counselor on two occasions in university (for exam stress) and was given sleeping medication which was effective; Mr. A drinks socially, doesn't smoke cigarettes and denies current or past substance abuse.

Medications   sulfasalazine 2 g p.o. daily; loperamide 2 mg caps p.o. prn; codeine phosphate 30 mg p.o. qid; over-the-counter sleeping pills

Medical History Other than having UC, Mr. A is healthy. In high school, he was knocked unconscious for under 10 seconds in a football game.

Personal/ Social History Mr. A was told he had an unremarkable birth. He met his developmental milestones appropriately. He attended school at age 5, which was age-appropriate. He did well in school and did not need remedial help at any point. He idealized one of his primary school teachers (a former athlete) and gives this as a partial reason for his occupation. Mr. A is exclusively heterosexual and began to date in late high school. Long-term relationships have been difficult for him — he describes his girlfriends as pushing him too much to leave his parents' house and make a commitment. He has never been married. Mr. A left home for one year of university and then sought employment only in his hometown. He describes himself as always trying to make his parents proud and felt they would be more interested and kept up to date on his progress if he lived in the same city.

Other than one speeding ticket, Mr. A has no current legal difficulties, and has never been charged with an offense. He has not been involved in military service.

Family History Mr. A is not aware of any members of his immediate family having been diagnosed with a psychiatric disorder. He recalls certain stress-related problems his father had, especially at times of union contract negotiations, and promotions. His extended family was similarly reported to be free of psychiatric difficulties as far as he knew.

Mental Status Exam
• Appearance — well groomed, wearing hospital pajamas
• Behavior — fidgeted and looked out the window at times, otherwise calm
• Speech/ Thought Form — no abnormalities detected (NAD)
• Thought Content — centered on school concerns and fear of surgery
• Affect & Mood — as described above
• Perception — NAD
• Insight & Judgment — deemed intact on the basis of his

awareness of his illness and appropriate actions to get help; he is willing to go along with the recommendations of his attending physician and listed the major long-term complications of UC and the risks of not receiving treatment
• Cognitive Functions — oriented x 3; registration, recent, and remote recall intact; general knowledge intact; concentration and attention as described

Summary Mr. A is a 32-year-old man admitted for a flare-up of UC, his 4th admission in 7 years. He relates the onset of a variety of mood and anxiety symptoms to the situation at work and the worsening of his physical state. He has a history of difficulty coping with situations that seem beyond his control and that may reflect negatively on him (especially tests and evaluations). Using DSM-IV criteria, he does not appear to have a major mood or anxiety disorder at this time.

Diagnostic Impression
Axis I: Adjustment Disorder With Mixed Anxiety and Depressed Mood
Axis II: Obsessive-Compulsive & Dependent Personality Traits
Axis III: Ulcerative Colitis
Differential Diagnosis: Depression, Generalized Anxiety Disorder

Treatment Recommendations for the Referring Team
• Suggest a TSH level & a folate level be drawn (due to sulfasalazine)
• A benzodiazepine (lorazepam 1mg or oxazepam 15mg) p.o. qhs can replace his sleeping medication (unknown at present)
• Given that he doesn't currently appear to have a clear-cut mood or anxiety disorder, a psychotropic medication is not indicated; agents useful in both these conditions (i.e. SSRIs & TCAs) can cause GI upset which may aggravate his condition and make it difficult to sort out whether it was his UC or the medication making him ill

• Because of the clear association between work-related stress and the seriousness of his flare-up, a complete resolution is advisable before he returns to work — suggest a medical leave of absence

Recommended Treatment by the C-L Team
• Mr. A is a suitable candidate for short-term psychotherapy which can begin this week if he is agreeable
• Our team will contact the school (with Mr. A's permission) to see if his performance has justifiably caused concern there

Reference
E.A. Walker, M.D. Gelfand, A.N. Gelfand, F. Creed & W. J. Katon
The Relationship of Current Psychiatric Disorder to Functional Disability and Distress in Patients with Inflammatory Bowel Disease
General Hospital Psychiatry 18(4): p. 220 — 229, 1996

Critique of the Three Notes

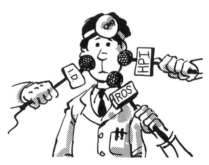

The medical note is a "bare bones" record of the admission outlining almost exclusively the physical aspects of the illness. There is a brief notation in the HPI and another in the physical exam section pertaining to the patient's emotional status. This is not an uncommon amount of documentation for a referral made early in the admission — the medical resident knew there was a need for a psychiatric consult.

The note by Dr. Froyd is a good, thorough, psychodynamically relevant document. Unfortunately, it misses the mark as a good consult note because several key areas are not addressed, even though the consult question is answered. This is a common pitfall among psychiatric residents (and consultants) who think 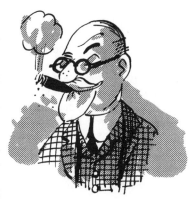 that the referring source is as interested in psychiatry as they are, and that every factoid of information should be included.

The note by Dr. Eager is a complete and satisfactory consult report. It embodies all of the elements discussed in this chapter though it is necessarily less detailed in certain areas than Dr. Froyd's note. Breaking down the various sections helps a busy physician identify which sections he or she would like to read. There is a thorough cataloging of diagnostic cri- 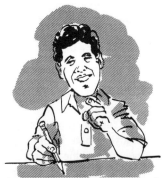 teria for the two conditions listed in the reason for referral. This not only illustrates the rationale for the diagnostic impression, it allows you to follow the progress of specific symptoms during your visits. Although there were few findings on the MSE, it was still performed and documented. Two features of medical relevance were discovered during the interview: the use of an over-the-counter sleeping medication and a distant head injury. The recommendations include consideration of biopsychosocial factors both for investigations and treatment. The suggested folate level was made after reading the particulars about this medication. The reference is from a psychiatry journal, not a medical one, which could be seen as implying that the referring source doesn't stay current with the literature. In some cases, the goals for psychotherapy may be omitted or given in more detail depending on confidentiality considerations and the interest of the referring source.

Summary

Psychiatric consultation reports answer two main questions:

- What is going on with the patient?
- What can be done about it?

A consult request in a sense forms a "contract" with explicit and implicit obligations. The consult note documents your opinion/answers to the above questions and outlines management suggestions. A suggested outline for reports is as follows:

- A clearly-written title, which includes your name, position, pager/ phone extension, and the referring source
- Time, date, length of interview; sources of information
- Identifying features of the patient
- A synopsis of the patient's medical illness and course
- Reason for the referral/ expectations of the consultee
- Outline of the biopsychosocial factors leading to the consult
- Detailed inquiry into factors related to the consult question
- Review of symptoms for other psychiatric illnesses
- Psychiatric history (including psychotherapy & medications)
- Medications, allergies, substance use

- Personal, social & family history; legal & military history
- Mental Status Examination
- Summary/ Impression/ Formulation with provisional and differential diagnoses
- Recommendations/ Suggestions
- References or articles

If the above list constitutes the "science" of writing a note, the "art" balances the following factors:

thorough documentation	vs.	interest level of the consultee
emphasis on detail	vs.	emphasis on confidentiality
technical jargon	vs.	precision in phenomenology
explaining rationale for recommendations	vs.	"just do it" approach
thorough investigations for physical causes	vs.	the expense and relatively low yield of abnormal results

References

S.A. Cohen-Cole, in
Consultation Psychitary: A Practical Guide
R. Michels, J.O. Cavenar & A.M. Cooper, Editors
Lippincott, Philadelphia, 1988

T.N. Garrick & N.L. Stotland
How To Write A Psychiatric Consultation
American Journal of Psychiatry 139(7): p. 849 — 855, 1982

R.C.W. Hall, E.R. Gardner, S.K. Stickney, A.F. LeCann et al
Physical Illness Manifesting as Psychiatric Illness
Archives of General Psychiatry 37: p. 989 — 995, 1980

C.F. McCartney, D.L. Evans & W. Richardson
Library Collection of the Psychosocial Publications in Consultation-Liaison Psychiatry
General Hospital Psychiatry 7(1): p. 73 — 82, 1985

M.L. Popkin, T.B. Mackenzie, R.C.W. Hall & A.L. Callies
Consultees' Concordance With Consultant's Psychotropic Drug Recommendations
Archives of General Psychiatry 37: p. 1017 — 1021, 1980

M.L. Popkin, T.B. Mackenzie, A.L. Callies et al
Yield of Psychiatric Consultants' Recommendations for Diagnostic Action
Archives of General Psychiatry 39: p. 843 — 845, 1982

M.L. Popkin, T.B. Mackenzie & A.L. Callies
Consultation-Liaison Outcome Evaluation
Archives of General Psychiatry 40: p. 215 — 219, 1983

N. L. Stotland & T.R. Garrick
Manual of Psychiatric Consultation
American Psychiatric Press, Inc. Washington, D.C., 1990

Z. Taintor, J. Spikes, L.H. Gise & J.J. Strain
Recording Psychiatric Consultations: A Preliminary Report
General Hospital Psychiatry 1(2): p. 139 — 149, 1979

4/ Implementing the Treatment Plan

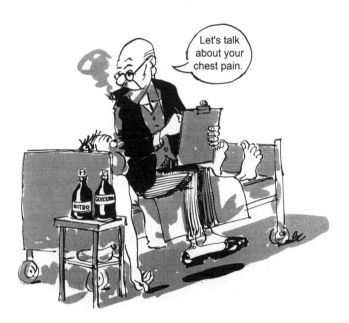

The two previous chapters have outlined the first four stages in the process of conducting a psychiatric consultation.

- **The Referral** (Ch. 2)
- **Preparing for the Consult** (Ch. 2)
- **Interviewing the Patient** (Ch. 2)
- **Writing the Consultation Report** (Ch. 3)
- **Implementing the Treatment Plan**

A thorough interview and a well-written note are two key factors in providing a psychiatric consultation. However, an appropriate or even elegant treatment plan doesn't benefit the patient until your recommendations are implemented by the referring source.

The degree to which consultees implement the recommendations in your treatment plan has been termed **concordance**. This chapter focuses the following areas:

- What level of concordance should be expected?
- Does the level of concordance vary with the type of recommendation made?
- Does the status of the person performing the consult make a difference?
- Why would consultees not implement recommendations?
- Do other specialist consultants have similar problems with concordance?
- What can be done to increase the degree of concordance?

Concordance

At this point in the consult process, you have taken care of the preliminary process matters outlined in the previous two chapters, interviewed the patient, and informed the referring source of your recommendations via your consult note. You may even have had an after-consult discussion with the consultee. You return the next day to check on the patient's progress and find that none of your suggestions have been implemented. You are not even sure if the primary physician has read your note. Your visit with the patient also reveals that the treating team made no mention of your plan at rounds.

Does this happen often? Is it you? Something you suggested? Or are they just getting around to your note and will give it due consideration when they have the chance? Should you contact the team to ask why, speak to a supervisor or colleague, or just wait it out? These and other salient matters will be dealt with in this section which reviews some of the literature on this topic.

Popkin, Mackenzie et al published a series of articles between 1979 and 1983 in a number of journals that explored various aspects of the implementation of psychiatric consultant's recommendations. They developed terminology that was used by other authors in subsequent articles:

> • **Concordance** was used to describe the degree of implementation of consult recommendations; the authors felt this term described the mutuality of the consultation interchange rather than the unilateral connotation of the term "compliance" (in this chapter concordance, compliance and implementation are used interchangeably)

> • **Representation** is the presence of the psychiatric diagnosis/ diagnoses on the medical discharge summary

The following sections summarize reports on various aspects of concordance with accompanying references. Because there are discrepancies between studies, for the sake of clarity and brevity, the emphasis here is on the positive findings (i.e. where something significant was found) from these reports.

CLOES

CLOES is an acronym for **Consultation-Liaison Outcome Evaluation System** and was developed by Popkin, Mackenzie et al. Their series of articles provides a set of standardized criteria to measure concordance. CLOES criteria are listed here in an abbreviated form to provide a frame. Criteria for **concordance (C)**, **partial concordance (PC)** and **nonconcordance (NC)** were developed to measure three major areas of study:

Compliance with psychotropic medication suggestions:
> • C — if started within 96 hours and the dosage was between 75 and 125% of that recommended
> • PC — if started within 96 hours and a dosage of between 50 to 74% or 126 to 150% of that recommended was used
> • NC — advised drug or equivalent not used within 96 hours in the absence of contraindications

Representation of consultants' psychiatric diagnoses:
> • C — if a verbatim or near-verbatim representation of the diagnosis was made
> • PC — an uncertain representation was made
> • NC — no mention of the diagnosis was made

Implementation of recommendations for diagnostic action
> • C — if the recommended action was implemented within 96 hours; if multiple recommendations were made and over 75% of them were carried out
> • PC — if multiple recommendations were made and

between 50 to 74% of them were followed
• NC — if the recommended action was not carried out, or in the case of multiple recommendations, less than 50% were carried out

In many studies, the PC category was re-scored or dropped from the analysis to gain a clearer appreciation for which variables were associated with C or NC outcomes. The criteria are fully listed in:

M.L. Popkin, T.B. Mackenzie & A.L. Callies
Consultation-Liaison Outcome Evaluation
Archives of General Psychiatry 40: p. 215 — 219, 1983

Concordance for Medication Recommendations

Popkin, Mackenzie et al began with a retrospective look at the degree of implementation for psychiatric consultant's medication suggestions. Their results were as follows:

• 200 consults were reviewed with psychotropic medication recommendations being made in 55% of cases
• Implementation was 68% C, 11% PC and 24% NC

They found that there were significant differences among the different actions involving medications, which were:

• Stop	93%
• Adjust	90%
• Continue (as taken prior to admission)	80%
• Start	68%

When a dosage was specified, concordance in starting medication was 68% vs. 46% when it was not. Overall, consultees started medications at 80% of the recommended dosage. A second study was conducted to determine related variables. They found statistically higher concordance levels where:

- A medication was either adjusted, continued or stopped (these actions formed a separate "non-start" group as the action of "starting" a medication has a lower concordance)
- Multiple recommendations were made
- The consult occurred in the first half of the admission
- The patient had a history of taking, or was currently using, a psychotropic medication
- The recommendation to start a medication was accompanied by a specified dosage (this was particularly so if the consultation note was shorter)

A study by Neill (1979) found that there were differences between types of recommended medications, with antipsychotics being concordant 90% of the time vs. 65% for benzodiazepines and 56% for tricyclic antidepressants. Huyse et al (1993) found that 77% of consults included a medication suggestion, and he concurred with the finding that medication recommendations made earlier in the hospital stay had a greater chance of implementation. Billowitz (1979) found that the referring service had differing compliance rates (with Medicine > Ob/Gyn > Surgery).

Summary for Medication Concordance

Referring physicians may exhibit a dichotomy in prescribing psychotropic medications in that they see a patient as someone who either would or would not use them. Previous or current use of psychotropics seems to make it easier for consultees to implement recommendations for drug treatments. The reason for referral may affect concordance in that psychotic or disruptive patients are more likely to be given medication.

Familiarity with psychotropic medication, or a higher degree of overlap between psychiatry and the referring specialty (e.g. Medicine > Surgery), increases concordance for medication suggestions.

The changing agendas during a patient's stay influence the timing of consult requests, as well as the receptiveness to medication suggestions.

References for Medication Concordance

A. Billowitz & W. Friedson
Are Psychiatric Consultants' Recommendations Followed?
Internat. J. of Psychiatry in Medicine 9(2): p. 179 — 189, 1978-9

F.J. Huyse, J.S. Lyons & J.J. Strain
The Sequencing of Psychiatric Recommendations
Psychosomatics 34: p. 307 — 313, 1993

J.R. Neill
Consultation Evaluation: I. Psychotropic Drug Recommendations
General Hospital Psychiatry April 1(1): p. 62 — 65, 1979

M.L. Popkin, T.B. Mackenzie, R.C.W. Hall & J.G. Garrard
Physicians' Concordance With Consultant's Recommendations for Psychotropic Medication
Archives of General Psychiatry 36: p. 386 — 389, 1979

M.L. Popkin, T.B. Mackenzie, R.C.W. Hall & A.L. Callies
Consultees' Concordance With Consultants' Psychotropic Drug Recommendations
Archives of General Psychiatry 37: p. 1017 — 1021, 1979

Concordance for Diagnostic Actions

Popkin (1980) reported that:

- In 29% of their consults, they suggested diagnostic action(s)
- The overall concordance for their cases was 53%

Then, he grouped the diagnostic actions into four subtypes and reported the concordance based on individual recommendations:

- Consultations (from other services)   67%
- Diagnostic procedures/exams   65%
- Laboratory determinations   61%
- Psychological testing   54%

The two most frequent recommendations in each category were respectively:

- Neurology & endocrinology (consultations)
- EEGs & EKGs (diag. procedures)
- Thyroid & other clinical chemistry tests (lab. tests)
- Personality & cognitive testing (psych. testing)

The difference in rates of concordance between these four groups was not statistically significant. Concordance was found to be higher in the following circumstances:

- As the age of the patient increased (especially > 60 years)
- With the diagnosis of an **organic mental disorder (OMD)**
- The longer the period of hospitalization after the consult
- With longer-term admissions

In a second study, Popkin (1982) looked at the prevalence of abnormal results for psychiatrists' diagnostic recommendations and found an overall yield of 45%. Patients with OMDs had the greatest likelihood of having an abnormal result (81%).

The tests with the highest yield of abnormal results were:

- MMPI   76%
- EEG   69%
- Thyroid function tests   52%
- Vitamin B_{12} level   47%
- Folate level   44%

Huyse (1993) reported concordance rates of 58% and 55% for biological diagnostic actions and psychosocial actions respectively which agrees with Popkin's results. Huyse's results indicated that psychosocial diagnostic actions were more likely to be implemented during an admission. In another study, Huyse (1990) found that diagnostic recommendations for actions that varied from the consultees' usual activities were less likely to be carried out. In particular, obtaining psychosocial information from general practitioners and families were the investigations with the lowest yields (40% and 52%). Popkin (1980) found that a follow-up note on the chart increased concordance.

Summary for Diagnostic Action Concordance

A consistent finding in these studies was a concordance rate of less than 60% for investigations, despite the relatively high yield of abnormal results when recommendations were implemented. Popkin (1982) suggested that once referring sources determine that a patient's problem is psychiatric, the evaluative process terminates.

Higher concordance rates later in an admission may be related to the complexity of the case and/or the perplexity of the consultee. Overall, referring sources are more interested in management recommendations than in evaluative ones.

References for Diagnostic Action Concordance

F.J. Huyse, J.J. Strain & J.S. Hammer
Interventions in C-L Psychiatry, Part II: Concordance
General Hospital Psychiatry 12: p. 221 — 231, 1990

F.J. Huyse, J.S. Lyons & J.J. Strain
The Sequencing of Psychiatric Recommendations
Psychosomatics 34: p. 307 — 313, 1993

M.L. Popkin, T.B. Mackenzie, & A.L. Callies
Consultees' Concordance With Consultants' Recommendations for Diagnostic Action
Journal of Nervous and Mental Disorders 168(1): p. 9 — 12, 1980

M.L. Popkin, T.B. Mackenzie, A.L. Callies & R.C.W. Hall
Yield of Psychiatric Consultants' Recommendations for Diagnostic Action
Archives of General Psychiatry 39: p. 843 — 845, 1982

Diagnostic Representation

Callies (1980) looked at the incorporation of psychiatric diagnoses (**representation**) in the medical/ surgical discharge summary from the initial consult note. After dropping PC cases from the evaluation, the overall concordance rate was 50%. Factors significantly related to concordance were:

- The primary medical diagnosis at discharge; if the patient's difficulties were deemed functional (psychiatric), the concordance rate increased to 79%
- The consultee's service; the results were broadly grouped into medical services (63%) and surgical services (11%)
- The number of days of hospitalization; concordant

cases were hospitalized fewer days at the time of the consult, spent fewer days in hospital after the consult, and had shorter overall admissions

In the 50% of cases that were NC, two-thirds made no mention of the diagnosis, while the other third contained inaccurate representations. Froese (1979) reported similar findings. The sample of cases used in Callies (1980) was combined with those from another period of evaluation and published by Popkin (1983). The combination of cases was examined and yielded an overall concordance of 52%. A more detailed analysis of consulting services revealed the following rates of concordance:

• Neurosurgery	59%
• Other	58%
• General Medicine	56%
• Neurology	54%
• Gynecology	29%
• General Surgery	21%

The variables found to be significant in Callies (1980) were confirmed in this expanded sample. In this study, diagnostic representation had the lowest concordance rate (52%) vs. 56% for diagnostic action and 69% for psychotropic drug recommendations.

In Popkin (1982), an assessment was made in randomly chosen cases as to whether the implemented diagnostic actions:

• Clarified or changed the conceptualization of the case by the consultee (23%)
• Made a contribution to ruling out a possible diagnosis or confirming an established or suspected one (73%)
• Were represented in the discharge summary (23%)

Summary for Diagnostic Representation

Since diagnosis is a pivotal factor in outlining a treatment plan, it is surprising that representation on discharge summaries rated the lowest level of concordance. With omissions occurring twice as often as inaccurate descriptions, psychiatric diagnoses are often not seen as relevant information. This can also reflect a lack of interest towards, or comprehension of, psychiatric nosology — particularly on surgical services. Tests recommended by consultants that led to a reconceptualization of a case were even less likely to receive mention. With longer admissions, the amount of information summarized on discharge reports may preclude mention of a psychiatric consultation. The low level of diagnostic representation highlights the need for a thorough examination of patients' charts for previous psychiatric consultations.

References for Diagnostic Representation

A.L. Callies, M.L. Popkin, T.B. Mackenzie & J. Mitchell
Consultees' Representation of Consultants' Psychiatric Diagnoses
American Journal of Psychiatry 137(10): p. 1250 — 1253, 1980

A.P. Froese
Is The Psychiatrist's Opinion Heard?
Internat. Journal of Psychiatry in Medicine 8: p. 295 — 301, 1977-78

M.L. Popkin, T.B. Mackenzie, A.L. Callies & R.C.W. Hall
Yield of Psychiatric Consultants' Recommendations for Diagnostic Action
Archives of General Psychiatry 39: p. 843 — 845, 1982

M.L. Popkin, T.B. Mackenzie, A.L. Callies & R.C.W. Hall
Consultation-Liaison Outcome Evaluation System
Archives of General Psychiatry 40: p. 215 — 219, 1983

Psychiatry vs. Cardiology Consult Outcomes

Mackenzie (1981), in a diversification move that would have made a burger chain proud, applied CLOES methodology to assess concordance rates in a sample of cardiology consults. Popkin (1981) compared the results from the above study to an equal number of psychiatric consults matched for hospital setting and time period. Frequency and concordance rates for medication and diagnostic action recommendations were compared. The results were as follows for medication recommendations:

- **Cardiac consults**
  frequency 49%   concordance 82%
- **Psychiatric consults**
  frequency 45%   concordance 69%

While the difference in concordance rates was statistically significant, the difference in frequency was not.

The results for diagnostic action recommendations were:

- **Cardiac consults**
  frequency 38%   concordance 73%
- **Psychiatric consults**
  frequency 29%   concordance 56%

There was a significant difference for both the rates of diagnostic recommendations and concordance between these groups. Popkin went on to elucidate the variables that were significant in determining the concordance for each type of recommendation and each service. The findings in this study did not vary from the positive findings outlined in the sections for medication recommendations and diagnostic actions for psychiatric consults.

The difference in concordance for medication recommendations was not found to be related to the identity of the consulting service. The factors relevant to concordance with cardiology consults had some overlap with those from psychiatry. When the type of drug recommendation was a "non-start" action (adjust, continue or stop) and multiple recommendations were made, concordance was higher for both services. The class of cardiac drug was a significant factor, which was not found in Popkin's results (though this was found to be an important factor in other studies). The factors that statistically increased concordance with diagnostic actions for cardiology consults were the presence of follow-up visits and the identity of the consult service. These factors were not the same in the psychiatry sample. The specific diagnostic action was unrelated to concordance in either group.

Summary for Comparing Consult Outcomes

This study found overall that concordance was higher for cardiology consultations. Different variables were important in determining the level of implementation between services.

References for Comparing Consult Outcomes

T.B. Mackenzie, M.L. Popkin, A.L. Callies et al
The Effectiveness of Cardiology Consultation
Chest 79: p. 16 — 22, 1981

M.L. Popkin, T.B. Mackenzie, A.L. Callies & J.N. Cohn
An Interdisciplinary Comparison of Consultation Outcomes
Archives of General Psychiatry 38: p. 821 — 825, 1981

The Psychiatrist as Consultee

Hall (1980) found that almost half of a series of one hundred psychiatric patients from lower socioeconomic classes had coexisting physical problems that either caused or affected their psychiatric symptoms sufficiently that admission was necessary. An additional one-third of these patients suffered from medical illnesses severe enough to require medical treatment.

Mackenzie (1983) investigated the outcome of medical-surgical consults on a psychiatric inpatient unit. This article was a more detailed study of referral outcomes than was provided in an earlier article by Bernstein (1980), who reported that 25% of their series of psychiatric patients received medical-surgical consults. Mackenzie found that 38% of the patients in his series received at least one consultation during their inpatient stay. The most common services involved were:

- Neurology 23%
- Gynecology 9%
- Endocrinology 9%

Additionally, three-quarters of all cardiology, endocrinology, and neurology consults were requested within the first two weeks of admission. Recommendation rates were as follows:

- Medication 27%
- Diagnostic action 46%

All of the consultations contained a diagnostic impression.

Concordance rates were as follows:

- Medication recommendations 79%
- Diagnostic action recommendations 75%
- Diagnostic representation 61%

Conducting Psychiatric Consultations — Explained

A summary of the Popkin and Mackenzie articles looking at concordance rates of psychiatric consults, medical-surgical consults to psychiatric units, and cardiology consults is as follows:

Frequency of Recommendations

	Consultant Psychiatrist[^]	Consultee Psychiatrist	Consultant Cardiologist[^]
Drug	45%	27%	49%
Diagnostic Action	29%	46%	38%

Concordance

	Consultant Psychiatrist[+]	Consultee Psychiatrist	Consultant Cardiologist[^]
Drug	63%	79%	82%
Diagnostic Action	53%	75%	73%
Diagnostic Representation	43%	61%	—

[^] results from Popkin (1981)
[+] results from Popkin (1983) using unadjusted rates

References for Psychiatrists as Consultees

R.A. Bernstein & D. Dreyfuss
Medical & Surgical Consultations to a General Hospital Psychiatry Unit
General Hospital Psychiatry 2: p. 267 — 270, 1980

R.C.W. Hall, E.R. Gardner, S.K. Stickney, A.F. LeCann & M.K. Popkin
Physical Illness Manifesting as Psychiatric Disease
Archives of General Psychiatry 37: p. 989 — 995, 1980

T.B. Mackenzie, M.L. Popkin, A.L. Callies & J. Kroll
Consultation Outcomes: The Psychiatrist as Consultee
Archives of General Psychiatry 40: p. 1211 — 1214, 1983

M.L. Popkin, T.B. Mackenzie, A.L. Callies & J.N. Cohn
An Interdisciplinary Comparison of Consultation Outcomes
Archives of General Psychiatry 38: p. 821— 825, 1981

M.L. Popkin, T.B. Mackenzie & A.L. Callies
Consultation-Liaison Outcome Evaluation System
Archives of General Psychiatry 40: p. 215 — 219, 1983

Other Positive Findings Regarding Concordance

"Positive findings" from other articles are listed in this section. By this, it is meant that the findings from studies having a significant effect on concordance are listed here. In many instances in the C-L literature, an article with certain findings can be negated by the findings of another. For example, where Popkin (1979) found that medication recommendations made in the first half of the admission had a higher concordance rate, Lanting (1984) found no such association. For this reason, the positive factors that had a bearing on concordance in at least one study are summarized to give a list of variables that *may* be important when considering concordance with your recommendations.

Lanting (1984) found that concordance for diagnostic action and representation was related to:

> • The reason for referral, with the highest levels of concordance being found when the consults involved substance abuse or investigating a possible psychogenic cause for physical problems
> • The type of referring service, with a rate of 60% for general medicine and 33% for general surgery

Huyse (1992) determined that the following factors were associated with increased concordance:

- The greater the number of recommendations
- A consultation performed earlier during the admission
- The higher the seniority/rank of the consultant

Huyse (1990) found the highest implementation rates for:

- Determining the timing of discharge (96%)
- Transferring care to another facility (95%)
- Using restraints (89%)
- Requesting other consultations (86%)
- Arranging outpatient care (86%)
- Increasing physical treatments (84%)

The lowest concordance rates in this study were for:

- Re-orienting cognitively impaired patients (21%)
- Obtaining information from the family doctor (40%)
- Providing objects to help re-orient patients (e.g. clock, newspapers, calendar) (48%)
- Obtaining information from the patient's family (52%)

Wise (1987) found that adjustment disorders and dysthymic disorders were the most likely to be omitted from discharge summaries. Neurosurgery and oncology referring sources were the most likely to omit psychiatric discharge diagnoses.

Wise (1987) also noted that 63% of patients' primary psychiatric diagnoses were missing from the admission note. Organic mental disorders, dementia, and substance abuse were the most likely conditions to be omitted.

References for Concordance Studies

F.J. Huyse, J.J. Strain & J.S. Hammer
Interventions in Consultation-Liaison Psychiatry
General Hospital Psychiatry 12: p. 221 — 231, 1990

F.J. Huyse, J.S. Lyons & J.J. Strain
Evaluating Psychiatric Consultations in the General Hospital
General Hospital Psychiatry 14: p. 363 — 369, 1992

R.H.H. Lanting & M.W. Hengeveld
Outcome of Psychiatric Consultation in a Dutch University Hosp.
Psychosomatics 25(8): p. 619 — 625, 1984

M.L. Popkin, T.B. Mackenzie, R.C.W. Hall & J.G. Garrard
Physicians' Concordance With Consultants' Recommendations For Psychotropic Medication
Archives of General Psychiatry 36: p. 386 — 389, 1979

T.N. Wise, L.S. Mann, R. Silverstein & J. Steg
CLOES: Resident or Private Attending Physicians' Concordance With Consultants' Recommendations
Comprehensive Psychiatry 28(5): p. 430 — 436, 1987

A Synthesis of Concordance Findings

As mentioned, it is difficult to define a coherent set of features that predict concordance for recommendations in an individual consultation. For this reason, the preceding sections have listed factors associated with positive outcomes in various studies, rather than providing a critical evaluation of each study.

A general finding from the C-L literature is that **process variables** are the most significant in determining concordance. For example, the timing of the consult during the admission, identity of the referring service, and age of the patient seem to have more to do with the implementation of recommendations than does the patient's medical problem, the patient's psychiatric diagnosis (other than OMD) or the seniority/ status of the consultant.

Local factors also play a large part in concordance. For example, Huyse (1992) was the only psychiatric consultant involved in his study, and he reported a special arrangement with the otolaryngology department (giving an overrepresentation of such patients). These "local factors" affect the study results to an extent that large differences in concordance are seen in the literature. For this reason, it is imperative to have an awareness of which of the factors listed (or not listed) are relevant to your service.

A second consistent principle from outcome studies is that consultees are more interested in recommendations involving patient management than in diagnostic evaluation. Huyse (1990) found the highest concordance for discharge recommendations, and other studies support the finding that these suggestions are almost always carried out.

While Popkin (1980) stated that a psychiatry consult is largely viewed as a nonmedical intervention, it also appears that referring sources prematurely end the medical investigation of patients with psychiatric symptoms. When OMD was diagnosed, concordance rose appreciably, in keeping with the medical model approach to understanding illness.

Concordance is higher with recommendations for single events with direct, tangible results that involve activities that are usually performed by consultees. For example, psychological management of patients on the ward and obtaining psychosocial information are less likely to be implemented.

Services having a greater overlap with psychiatry are more likely to implement recommendations and record discharge diagnoses. This has a particular relevance to surgical services, who consistently rated the lowest in these areas. The timing of consult requests is an important factor, but has two aspects. Early requests may indicate:

- A greater appreciation for psychosocial issues
- That the medical management is not yet firmly established and the consultee is more open to your input

Early requests also have the practical advantage that there is a longer time period in which recommendations can be implemented. On the other hand, consult recommendations involving patients with longer-term hospital stays or complex situations are also associated with higher levels of implementation. While there is some debate, making multiple recommendations appears to increase concordance, possibly because this indicates your active involvement in the patient's care.

References for Concordance

F.J. Huyse, J.J. Strain & J.S. Hammer
Interventions in Consultation-Liaison Psychiatry
General Hospital Psychiatry 12: p. 221 — 231, 1990

F.J. Huyse, J.S. Lyons & J.J. Strain
Evaluating Psychiatric Consultations in the General Hospital
General Hospital Psychiatry 14: p. 363 — 369, 1992

M.L. Popkin, T.B. Mackenzie & A. L. Callies
Consultees' Concordance With Consultants' Recommendations for Diagnostic Action
Journal of Nervous and Mental Disorders 168(1): p. 9 — 12, 1980

Why Would Consultees Not Implement Recommendations?

As outlined previously, the biases that influence requests for psychiatric consultation continue to make an impact on the implementation of recommendations. Some of these factors apply to consults in general, while others apply to psychiatric consults specifically.

Factors that Apply to Consults in General

• Unfortunately, some consultants reinforce their "expert" status by making recommendations that are poorly conceived, not essential, and may even be unhelpful

• Recommendations may be poorly explained or deemed not pertinent to the patient's care; additionally, consultees may lack the skills to perform certain actions (e.g. a thorough MSE)

• The cost involved in implementing tests is a factor, though Popkin (1981) found that more expensive procedures were more likely to be carried out

• Representation may be deficient because physicians are taught to be conservative with their diagnoses and to search for a single condition which explains all of a patient's symptoms; in cases of serious illness, it may seem sufficient to record that the patient survived and list only the factors directly related to the physical aspects of recovery

Lee (1983) found complete disagreement between consultant and consultee regarding the reason for referral (principal clinical issue) in 14% of cases. In these situations, there was significantly less usefulness attributed to the consult in assisting with diagnosis or management. Although this study did not monitor concordance, it is likely that the implementation of recommendations was lower when the consult wasn't perceived as being helpful. Interestingly, house officers rated an average of 7% of the consults they requested as being either "superfluous" or "for educational value only" even when there was agreement on the reason for consultation.

Factors Specific to Psychiatric Consultations

• Of all the medical specialties, psychiatry has the greatest range of reasons for which consultation is requested; if the referring source is seeking help with patient management, recommendations for diagnostic action may be seen as being beyond the scope of the consultation

• The request for a psychiatric consult may be a signal to indicate the end of the patient's organic investigation

• If referring sources have made an oversight, it may be less palatable to have a psychiatric service discover this than someone else

• Psychiatry may not be viewed as being scientific enough, or that a psychiatric diagnosis is nothing more than a subjective opinion; the diagnostic rationale and nosology are less likely to be understood by non-psychiatric physicians who may be uncomfortable with merely echoing the impression from the consult note

• One of the most enduring pieces of information physicians retain about psychiatric medications is that they can cause a diverse number of side effects; consultees may be reluctant to start psychotropic medications for fear that this could interfere with existing medical treatments or cause complications that will prolong the patient's stay (e.g. neuroleptic malignant syndrome)

• Consultees may be seeking affirmation that the

patient presents a challenging case and that they require reassurance that they're doing a thorough job; in a related instance, occasionally a **negative consult** is sought, in which the referring source seeks assurances that nothing has been missed or that nothing more can be done for the patient

• Local or process aspects may apply, resulting in an arbitrary degree of concordance; while these factors are largely beyond the consultees' control, it is still important to be aware of them, and to periodii cally let referring sources know that you are monitoring the effectiveness of your recommendations

Is There An Optimum Level of Concordance?

In Mackenzie (1983), psychiatrists didn't completely implement management suggestions when requesting consults. Rather, concordance was found to be 79% for drug recommendations and 75% for diagnostic actions. Popkin (1981) found that cardiologists enjoyed concordance rates of 82% for treatment recommendations and 73% for diagnostic actions. These rates are an important guide because there is less of a disparity in the expertise in physical medicine between consultant and consultee in these cases.

Lee (1983) studied house officers' perceptions of the value of a consultation for the purpose of diagnosis and management. He found that 77% were rated as either crucial, contributory or confirmatory for diagnosis and 82% for management. In cases where there is agreement on these matters, the referring team is much more likely to implement suggestions.

Pooling these findings, it appears that concordance rates of between 75% to 85% are what our colleagues are achieving.

A concordance rate of 100% is not obtainable in hospitals where recommendations must be approved before they can be implemented. For clinical and legal reasons, primary physicians retain control of their patients' management and do not turn it over to the various consultants whom they ask for advice. Discretion in implementing suggestions indicates that consultees critically review the care they provide for their patients, and that consults are one aspect of this process.

Summary of Nonconcordance Findings

Popkin (1980) noted that the implementation rates were not related to the type of diagnostic action recommended. Because there was as much resistance to recommendations for psychological testing as there was to other investigations, he felt the disinterest was not based on psychiatrists' competence in requesting tests. Rather, he stated that *"the phenomenon seems to be a disinclination engendered by the very act of seeking a psychiatric consultation."*

The studies discussed in this chapter reveal significantly higher concordance rates for cardiology consults. The degree of concordance shown by psychiatrists when requesting consults was very close to that obtained by the cardiologists. Based on the findings of the studies presented in this chapter, it appears that psychiatric C-L services face unique difficulties regarding concordance. The biases that exist against even requesting consults continue to exert an influence that limits the implementation of recommendations and ultimately the usefulness of psychiatric interventions.

References for Nonconcordance Findings

T. Lee, E.M. Pappius & L. Goldman
Impact of Inter-Physician Communication on the Effectiveness of Medical Consultations

The American Journal of Medicine 74: p. 106 — 112, 1983
T.B. Mackenzie, M.L. Popkin, A.L. Callies & J. Kroll
Consultation Outcomes: The Psychiatrist As Consultee
Archives of General Psychiatry 40: p. 1211— 1214, 1983

M.L. Popkin, T.B. Mackenzie, & A.L. Callies
Consultees' Concordance With Consultants' Recommendations for Diagnostic Action
Journal of Nervous and Mental Disorders 168(1): p. 9 — 12, 1980

M.L. Popkin, T.B. Mackenzie & A.L. Callies
Improving the Effectiveness of Psychiatric Consultation
Psychosomatics 22(7): p. 559 — 563, 1981

M.L. Popkin, T.B. Mackenzie, A.L. Callies & J.N. Cohn
An Interdisciplinary Comparison of Consultation Outcomes
Archives of General Psychiatry 38: p. 821 — 825, 1981

Strategies to Improve Concordance

Studies have consistently found that process and local variables are more important than clinical variables in determining concordance. Consultants need to be aware of interventions that will increase concordance by altering the consultation process.

Recommendations
- Where multiple recommendations are made, list the most important one(s) first
- Wise (1987) found that the number of recommendations averaged between 1—3 for the consult note and initial note and 1—2 on follow-up visits
- Use a clearly demarcated section of your consult report to list recommendations
- Be specific and be brief
- Be decisive; avoid conditional suggestions
- Keep concordance rates in mind; explain your rationale for recommendations you know are less likely to be implemented

Follow-up Visits
- Sensky (1986) reported that for two-thirds of consult patients, only two visits were made
- Making follow-up visits and leaving progress notes has been correlated with increasing concordance (use these visits to remind referring sources about your suggestions)
- Following patients conveys your interest and allows you to evaluate the effectiveness of your interventions
- If primary physicians are aware you are monitoring concordance, it may increase

Assign Responsibility
- Interventions are best made by specific people
- Contract with consultees regarding who will carry out your recommendations
- The more the intervention departs from the person's usual activities, the less likely it is to be implemented
- You may need to teach others (or arrange for instruction) the first time a task is performed

Structure Your Approach
- Use reminders
- Tailor the treatment to fit the referring source
- introduce components sequentially where possible
- Monitor the results personally
- Provide positive feedback to the consultees

Ask About Nonconcordance
- Popkin allowed 96 hours for implementation; the first and last 24 hours of an admission are time periods where compliance is likely to be low
- Ask consultees about their rationale for not

implementing your recommendations — it is the
only way you will discover the local and process
variables operating with that referring source at
your hospital
• Because a degree of nonconcordance is
expected, approach the problem as an intellectual
curiosity, not as a comment on your ability

Guggenheim (1978) said "*the inexperienced consultant places little emphasis on selling suggestions to the consultee and does not try to overcome the mild suspicion with which consultees often regard consultations of all specialties.*"

References for Improving Concordance

F. Guggenheim
A Marketplace Model of Consultation Psychiatry
American J. of Psychiatry 135(11): p. 1380 — 1383, 1978

R.B. Haynes, D.W. Taylor & D.L. Sackett
Compliance in Health Care
Johns Hopkins University Press, Baltimore, 1979

T. Sensky
The General Hospital Psychiatrist: Too Many Tasks And Too Few Roles?
British Journal of Psychiatry 148: p. 151 — 158, 1986

T.N. Wise, L.S. Mann, R. Silverstein & J. Steg
CLOES: Resident or Private Attending Physicians' Concordance With Consultants' Recommendations
Comprehensive Psychiatry 28(5): p. 430 — 436, 1987

Ten Commandments (C-L Version)

- Determine the question
- Establish urgency
- Look for yourself
- Be as brief as appropriate
- Be specific
- Provide contingency plans
- Honor thy turf (or thou shalt not covet thy neighbor's patient)
- Teach. . . with tact
- Talk is cheap. . . and effective
- Follow-up

L. Goldman, T. Lee & P. Rudd
Ten Commandments For Effective Consultations
Archives of Internal Medicine 143: p. 1753 — 1755, 1983
© American Medical Association, Used with permission

Ten More Commandments

- Thou shalt love thy fellow physician as thyself
- Thou shalt not procrastinate
- Thou shalt not obfuscate
- Thou shalt be concrete
- Thou shalt honor thy patient's spouse, children, and parents
- Thou shalt not hibernate
- Thou shalt persevere
- Thou shalt not preach
- Thou shalt not steal thy fellow physician's patients
- Thou shalt not shirk thy duty to thy hospital medical staff or thy local medical society

R.O. Pasnau
Ten Commandments of Medical Etiquette for Psychiatrists
Psychosomatics 26(2): p. 128 — 132, 1985
© American Psychiatric Press, Inc., Used with permission

Other Concordance References

F.J. Huyse, J.J. Strain & J.S. Hammer
Interventions in Consultation-Liaison Psychiatry, Part I: Patterns of Recommendations
General Hospital Psychiatry 12: 213 — 220, 1990

T.B. Karasu, R. Plutchik, H. Conte, B. Siegel et al
What Do Physicians Want From A Psychiatric Consultation Service?
Comprehensive Psychiatry 18: p. 73 — 81, 1977

A.J. Krakowski
Psychiatric Consultation in the General Hospital: An Exploration of Resistances
Diseases of the Nervous System 36: p. 242 — 244, 1975

T.B. Mackenzie, M.K. Popkin & A.L. Callies
CLOES, Part I: Teaching Applications
J.of Nervous and Mental Dis. 169(10): p. 648 — 653, 1981

K.R. Özbayrak
Concordance: Sequencing of Psychiatric Recommendations (letter)
Psychosomatics 35(2): p. 171 — 172, 1994

T.L. Thompson II, T.N. Wise & A.B. Kelley et al
Improving Psychiatric Consultation to Non-Psychiatric Physicians
Psychosomatics 31: p. 80 — 84, 1990

S.J. Schleifer, S. Bhardwaj, A. Lebovits et al
Predictors of Physician Nonadherence to Chemotherapy Regimens
Cancer 67: p. 945 — 951, 1991

C. van Dyke, D. Rice, P. Pallett & H. Leigh
Psychiatric Consultation: Compliance and Level of Satisfaction With Recommendations
Psychother. Psychosom. 33: p. 14 — 24, 1980

The Consultation Process

Obtain the following information at the time the consultation is requested:

"I'M SURE"

The Referral

Identifying Factors
Medical Problem(s)

Source of Referral
Urgency
Reason for Referral
Expectations of the Consultee

Preparing for the Consult

Consider the four entities involved in the consultation:
• Patient
• Consultee
• Reason for Referral
• C-L Service

Before seeing the patient:
• Refresh your knowledge of the medical/ surgical illness
• Contact the ward
• Read the chart

Interviewing the Patient

The C-L Interview:
• Explain the purpose and limitations of the interview
• Spend time developing rapport by discussing the physical illness
• Try to find a private area to conduct the interview
• Your priority is to answer the consultation question
• Be flexible in your interview style

The Consult Note

• Title, date, time, duration
• Your name, rank and phone #
• List sources of information

• Relevant personal information about the patient and a synopsis of the medical/ surgical problem
• Restate (or state) the purpose for the consultation and the expectations of the consultee

• A pertinent history incorporating biopsychosocial factors
• Eliciting symptoms and distillation of a diagnostic impression
• A personal history including reactions to stress and illness, substance use, legal problems, etc.

• Screening questions to search for comorbid conditions
• List significant negatives
• Perform an MSE on all patients

• Provide an impression, summary or formulation
• List the impediments in obtaining information (if any)
• Sign your note

Implementing Recommendations

• Develop a biopsychosocial management plan involving investigations, short, and longer term treatments
• Clearly indicate who should be making the above interventions
• Speak to consultees directly about urgent concerns
• Monitor concordance

From *Sigmundocopy, The Bases*
by David J. Robinson M.D., © Rapid Psychler Press

The Author

Dave Robinson is a psychiatrist practicing in London, Ontario, Canada. His particular interests are consultation-liaison psychiatry and both undergraduate and postgraduate education. He is a graduate of the University of Toronto Medical School and is a Lecturer in the Department of Psychiatry at the University of Western Ontario in London, Canada.

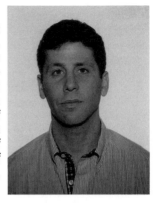

The Artist

Brian Chapman is a resident of Oakville, Ontario, Canada. He was born in Sussex, England and moved to Canada in 1957. Brian was formerly a Creative Director at Mediacom. He continues to freelance and is versatile in a wide range of media. He is a master of the caricature, and his talents are constantly in demand.

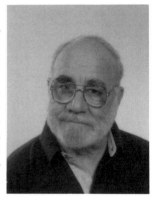

Rapid Psychler Press

Rapid Psychler Press was founded in 1994 with the aim of producing textbooks and resource materials that further the use of humor in mental health education. In addition to textbooks, Rapid Psychler Press specializes in producing slides and overheads for presentations.